SOUL MAGIC

Ancient Wisdom for Modern Mystics

Arizona Bell and Morgan Garza

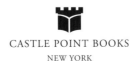

CASTLE POINT BOOKS

NEW YORK

www.castlepointbooks.com

The Castle Point Books trademark is owned by Castle Point Publishing, LLC. Castle Point books are published and distributed by St. Martin's Press.

ISBN 978-1-250-25304-0 (hardcover)
ISBN 978-1-250-25305-7 (ebook)

Design by Melissa Gerber

Our books may be purchased in bulk for promotional, educational, or business use. Please contact your local bookseller or the Macmillan Corporate and Premium Sales Department at 1-800-221-7945, extension 5442, or by email at MacmillanSpecialMarkets@macmillan.com.

First Edition: 2020

10 9 8 7 6 5 4 3 2 1

CONTENTS

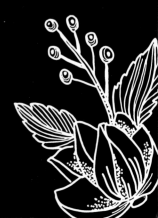

"Wonder is the
beginning
of wisdom."

—*Socrates*

INTRODUCTION

In the modern age where everyone including Aunt Sally is a "guru," the many paths to wisdom that are promoted by endless spiritual advisors can feel overwhelming and contradictory. They can even be more harmful than helpful. On our own personal spiritual quests, we've found that ancient wisdoms (paired with our own fine-tuned intuition) are the soul's true magic. They are the holy grail of spiritual and personal development.

In our weekly podcast *Spirit Guides Radio*, we aim to be a modern voice for these tried-and-true ancient wisdoms in which we so firmly believe. Each week, we have in-depth conversations with respected spiritual teachers and healers who shed light on the ins and outs of all things spiritual. Through this exploration of our own souls' magic and the inspired work that we do every day, we have compiled this guide to what we consider to be the most profound and relevant ancient self-healing methods for modern mystics.

With the onslaught of new, and often unproven, spiritual theories and self-help advice out there, looking to the trusted techniques of our ancestors is the surest path forward. These modalities have stood the test of time because their potency and healing power are irrefutable, spanning time, space, and cultures. They have endured because *they work*, and when we invest in learning such timeless wisdom, our lives begin to work, too.

There are many personal development modalities with deep roots in the ancient past that are still vibrantly alive in the modern world. As you explore this book through the lens of your own unique soul, remember that this is not a stringent to-do list, but a reliable map to guide you through the ups and downs of your ever-expanding spiritual path. Don't feel pressured to do it all. Just choose a modality (or five!) that calls to you, and dive in. If you find that something feels overwhelming or unappealing, skip it. Alternatively, if you were into one thing for a while and then find that it's suddenly not doing it for you anymore, drop it. There are no rules except to invest your time in what lights you up!

You are your own guru, and the point of any serious spiritual path is to be true to your highest self. At its core, *spirituality is about being authentic*, and all the techniques in this book are lighthouses to help you find your innate authenticity in a social age where being true to your uniqueness isn't always celebrated. This is your permission slip to do what feels in alignment with where you are right now and where you want to go. Simply choose your flavor, follow your intuition, and make changes when called to do so, allowing it to be a prescription that evolves as your life does.

In the profound words of French philosopher Albert Camus: "You will never be able to experience everything. So, please, do poetical justice to your soul and simply experience yourself." That's what this book is for: to guide you on your journey to experiencing your most soulful, magical, mystical self.

With endless distractions and to-do lists, not to mention the complicated world events that throw us off balance, it can be difficult to feel connected to the world around and within. On the one hand, social media has us feeling more connected than ever, yet many experts say that, particularly in the West, we are collectively suffering from loneliness and a feeling of disconnection. Disconnection is nothing more than a spiritual disease that must be healed by spiritual solutions. By studying and integrating the ancient practices outlined in this book, you are taking the first steps to plug back into your soul, awaken your self-healing power, and remember the truth that we are all connected.

No matter which modalities speak to your soul, please remember that the source of healing is always you! True spiritual connection and healing are found right inside each of us—we just need to know where to look. The ancient techniques in this book point the way to your own brand of "soul magic." By listening to the wonder of your soul, the path to wisdom will be cleared for you.

Love, light, and black holes,
Arizona Bell and Morgan Garza

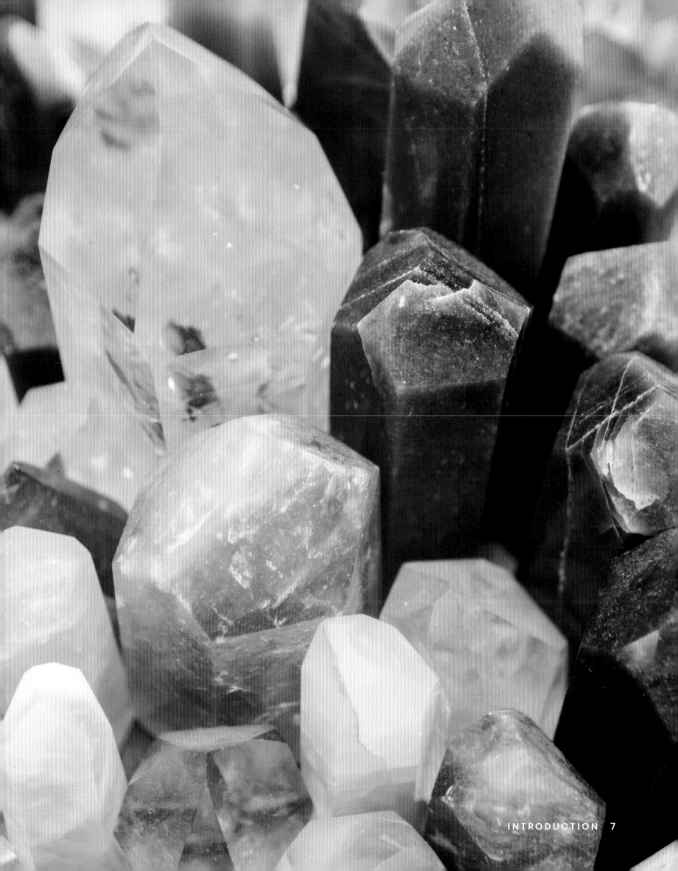

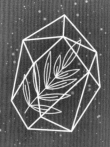

PART 1

NATURE MAGIC

————— ••• —————

Nature magic is the first magic. It's our most primitive of musings. Within this organic foundation, numerous ways of healing grow from soil into spirit. When we turn to nature, whether it's communing with plants' innate healing properties or crystals' divine energetic structures, we are also looking within. And it's in that inward journey where we gain the most perspective on our sacred origin, our special place in the world, and our active role in our health and vitality.

Humanity spent millennia conversing with plants, cataloging scents, harnessing the power of crystals, and unlocking the deepest secrets of the universe. As modern mystics, we continue to look to nature in times of distress. Somewhere deep down, we know that nature is our biggest ally for self-reflection, self-healing, and self-empowerment.

————— ••• —————

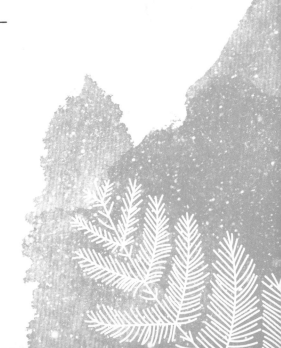

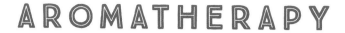

AROMATHERAPY

"Healing begins with an aromatic bath and daily massage."

—Hippocrates

Imagine the scent of bread baking in a warm kitchen, or pine needles crushed underfoot as you hike through the woods, or a freshly picked rose from your grandmother's garden. Did you smell them? Did they evoke feelings of nostalgia or childhood memories? This is your brain on aromatherapy.

Aromatherapy—the use of aromatic plant extracts and essential oils for healing and cosmetic purposes—has deep roots in human history. From Egypt to China and everywhere in between, for thousands of years, plant extracts in the form of essential oils and incense have been used by our ancestors for natural healing and spiritual expansion.

Ancient Egyptians were using aromatherapy in their daily lives and created aromatherapy blends for every possible need. For many centuries in the ancient world, essential oils were the only remedies for widespread diseases and conditions. Interestingly, during the infamous Black Plague, very few people who worked in the perfume and glove industries (where these oils were used abundantly) became ill.

Despite its rich ancient history, all forms of herbal medicine more or less disappeared until French chemist and scholar René-Maurice Gattefossé resuscitated the art in the 1920s. Known today as the father of aromatherapy, Gattefossé rediscovered the lost virtues of aromatherapy by accident while working in the lab of the cosmetics firm owned and named after his family (which is still in business today!). Legend has it that he burned his hand severely during an experiment and instinctively plunged his hand into the closest tub of liquid, which happened to be lavender essential oil. His burn healed impressively fast and with very little scarring, thus beginning his intense interest in essential oils. Today, aromatherapy is once again becoming a common and effective healing practice.

"Plants are remedies: for empty souls, meaningless lives, and generationally wounded bodies."

—*Jane Mayer*, THE CALL OF THE PLANTS: A BEGINNER'S GUIDE TO PLANT MEDICINE

Essential Oils

The abundant plants on our beautiful planet contain compounds that can't be seen with the naked eye. These compounds are hidden within the roots, flowers, seeds, bark, resin, leaves, or other areas of the plant, and they are the source of essential oils. Essential oils are what give a plant its aroma as well as protect it from insects and tough environmental conditions. **Because they are highly concentrated, essential oils are extremely potent and, therefore, have profound healing capabilities, both physically and spiritually.** In order for us to use them, though, they need to be distilled.

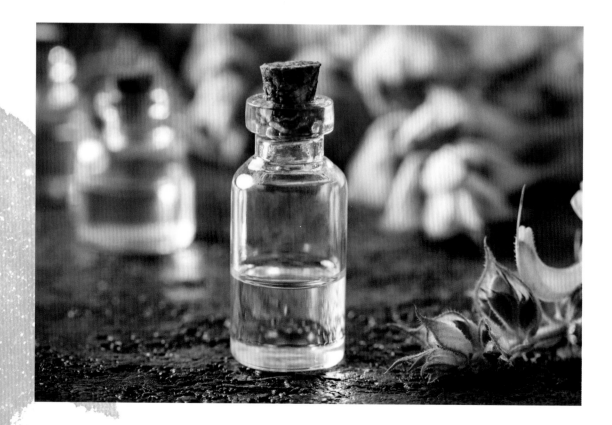

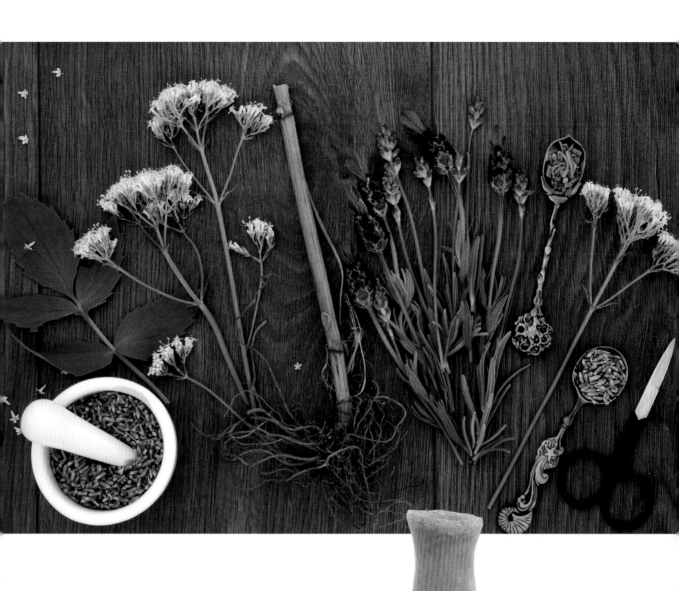

Because it takes copious amounts of plant matter to create essential oils, they should be used consciously and with reverence.

WAYS TO USE ESSENTIAL OILS

Because essential oils are absorbed through the skin, they're commonly used as additives in body oils, creams, lotions, clay masks, and hot and cold compresses. (Never ingest them or apply them "neat" or undiluted to your skin; they should always be added to some kind of carrier oil or other product.) These oils can also be added to bathwater and to facial steamers, so you can both inhale the scent and absorb it into your skin. Adding essential oils to aromatic spritzers allows you to spray your home, purify the air, calm your emotions during times of tension, or induce sleepiness. Lavender essential oils, for example, are commonly sprayed on sheets and pillows to set you on a smooth path to dreamland.

Essential oil diffusers are another convenient and refreshing way to experience the potent power of essential oils in your daily life. The scent of the oil or oil blend wafts through the air and works its healing magic on all who come into contact with it, bringing the calming effect of aromatherapy to your home or work environment. Try diffusing jasmine for reducing anxiety during the workday. Unlike other calming oils, it relaxes the nervous system without causing sleepiness.

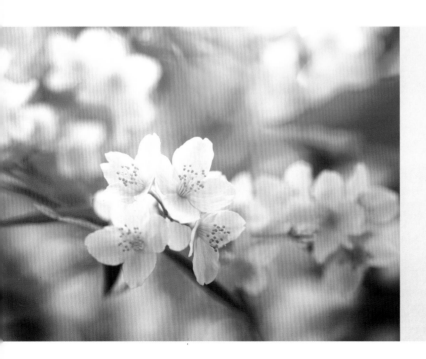

Pure, Simple, and Safe

Always buy your essential oils from a reputable supplier and make sure they do not contain additives or synthetic ingredients but are 100 percent essential oil. Please do your research first, as some essential oils are toxic in high quantities.

THREE ESSENTIAL OILS FOR SELF-HEALING

Essential oils are powerful allies for physical and spiritual healing. Here are our top three oils that can support your body's natural healing system.

ROSEMARY

You may be familiar with the taste of rosemary as a culinary herb, but did you know that rosemary also has numerous physical and spiritual healing properties? A relatively inexpensive essential oil with antiseptic qualities, rosemary has been used for centuries in sickrooms and hospitals. Physically, rosemary is known to stimulate hair growth, strengthen memory, and increase circulation.

Rosemary's spiritual healing strengths are similarly potent and can be used for cleansing space, encouraging peace of mind, emotional release, and psychic purification. Rosemary also aids in psychic development *and* psychic protection. Rosemary oil can be inhaled or applied topically. It is very concentrated, so use only a few drops at a time.

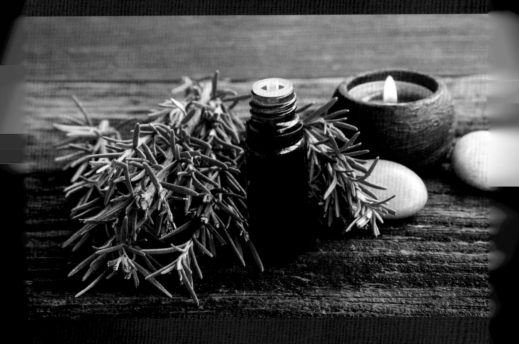

"Where rosemary grows, the woman rules the house."

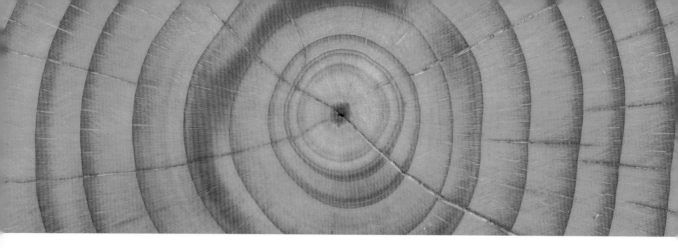

CEDAR

Cedar: It's not just for closets! Lebanese cedarwood was used to construct the Temple of King Solomon, cedar resin was used to embalm Egyptian mummies, and cedarwood is considered sacred to the Cherokee Native Americans. The magical properties of this essential oil cannot be stressed enough!

On a physical level, because it is antifungal, antiseptic, and anti-inflammatory, this woodsy-scented oil is a great helper for many health issues, especially those related to the skin (goodbye, acne!) and hair. And if mosquitos give you too much attention, you can use cedar oil as an effective bug repellent.

When used in aromatherapy, cedarwood has sedative qualities and greatly helps those who suffer from insomnia. Additionally, cedarwood is the perfect essential oil to help create a sacred space for grounding on your spiritual path.

SANDALWOOD

Sandalwood has long been associated with mysticism and has been one of the main scents burning in temples. This essential oil has a special constituent called *sesquiterpene*, which directly stimulates the pineal gland, where our third eye is found, and invokes a higher state of consciousness, bringing us into a state of deep openness where inspiration and inner guidance can be more easily received.

Sandalwood oil has numerous physical benefits as well and has long been used to prevent wrinkles and other signs of aging, to treat many skin conditions, from rashes to acne, and to promote wound healing.

POPULAR ESSENTIAL OILS AND THEIR USES

The following is a list of the most popular essential oils according to the National Association for Holistic Aromatherapy.

ESSENTIAL OIL	USES
Clary sage	Relieves menstrual cramps, aphrodisiac, relaxing, relieves stress and anxiety, used to manage pain in labor
Cypress	Astringent, relieves muscle spasms and pain, treats respiratory problems, relieves edema, helps cellulitis
Eucalyptus	Expectorant, decongestant, clears the mind, energizing, helpful for cold and flu season
Fennel	Digestive, antimicrobial, helps menstrual irregularities
Geranium	Useful for PMS and hormonal imbalance, antimicrobial, relieves nerve pain
Ginger	Digestive, relieves gas and constipation, treats nausea, anti-inflammatory, relieves pain, warming
Helichrysum	Helps regenerate cells, heals wounds, anti-inflammatory, helps with bruising and swelling
Lavender	Calming, relieves anxiety, heals wounds and burns, treats itchiness from insect bites, good for skin care because it helps with cell regeneration
Lemon	Antimicrobial, antioxidant, uplifting, relieves stress, cleansing, enhances immune system
Lemongrass	Cleansing, antiviral, repels insects, antimicrobial
Neroli	Relieves anxiety and PMS, antidepressant, relieves muscle cramps, nourishing
Patchouli	Anti-inflammatory, antidepressant, soothes the nervous system
Peppermint	Relieves nausea, helps with muscle pain and spasms, relieves headaches, energizing
Roman chamomile	Relieves menstrual cramps, sedative, relieves anxiety and stress, treats insomnia, anti-inflammatory
Rose	Helps regenerate cells, aphrodisiac, relieves menstrual cramps, relieves anxiety and stress, treats PMS
Rosemary	Relieves respiratory and sinus congestion from colds and flu, clears the mind, stimulates circulation
Tea tree	Antimicrobial, antifungal, antiviral, antibacterial
Vetiver	Calming, grounding, astringent
Ylang-ylang	Aphrodisiac, antidepressant, nourishing, relieves muscle cramps

Incense

"Light the incense! You have to burn to be fragrant."

—Rumi

The ancient Egyptians weren't burning incense every single day in their temples just because it smelled nice! Incense was considered so spiritually powerful that they even had a god of incense and aromatherapy, Nefertum. In biblical times, the three wise men brought the valuable and symbolic gifts of frankincense and myrrh for the baby messiah. In ancient China, buildings were built *solely* for incense ceremonies. And the Native Americans' use of sage incense for purification purposes is well known.

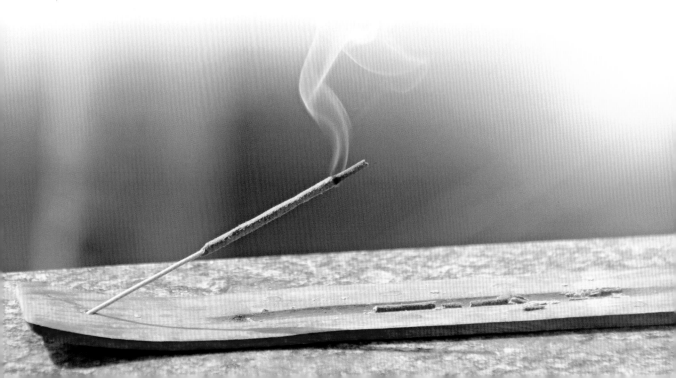

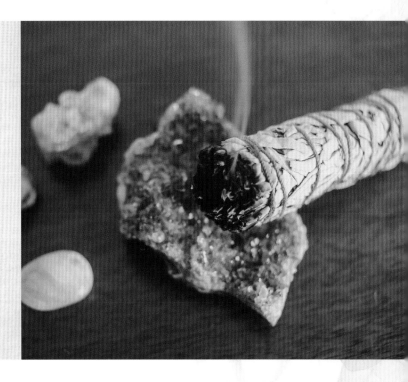

> One day while walking in the woods, I came upon some pine trees and was immediately overcome with nostalgia for the summer camp I went to as a kid. It seemed that right in front of me I could see the path leading from the main lodge to the cabins and I felt a strong longing for that time. Kicking up the scent of pine needles that day created an intense and poignant memory.
>
> —Alex, 43

As early as the 7th century BC, there was even an incense trade route referred to as the "Incense Road," which provided a network of land and sea routes whose main purpose was to carry Arabian frankincense and myrrh. In nearly every ancient culture in the world, burning incense was central to spiritual worship because people knew that scents could transport humans to higher spiritual planes.

We all can intuit the power of smell by recalling a time when we have been brought back to a good memory from our past just by inhaling a certain scent. That's because the sense of smell is closely connected to the limbic system, the place in our brains that plays a major role in mood, memory, and emotion.

Beyond merely prompting us to recall good times, scents also can move us beyond reason and help us leave our overactive minds and tune in to our underrepresented hearts. **The right scents can unlock higher spiritual realms within us.**

FRANKINCENSE

At one time, frankincense, a resin derived from the Boswellia tree, was worth more than silver and gold. That's how powerful it is! Burning frankincense has long symbolized prayer rising to the heavens, making frankincense a favorite cross-cultural tool for attuning with the divine. It is considered an extremely potent ally for spiritual cleansing.

There are plenty of ways in which frankincense can do your body, mind, and soul good. In addition to being a natural antidepressant, frankincense has anti-inflammatory, antiseptic, and astringent properties, and it is beneficial to people suffering from asthma, rheumatoid arthritis, Crohn's disease, osteoarthritis, and collagenous colitis.

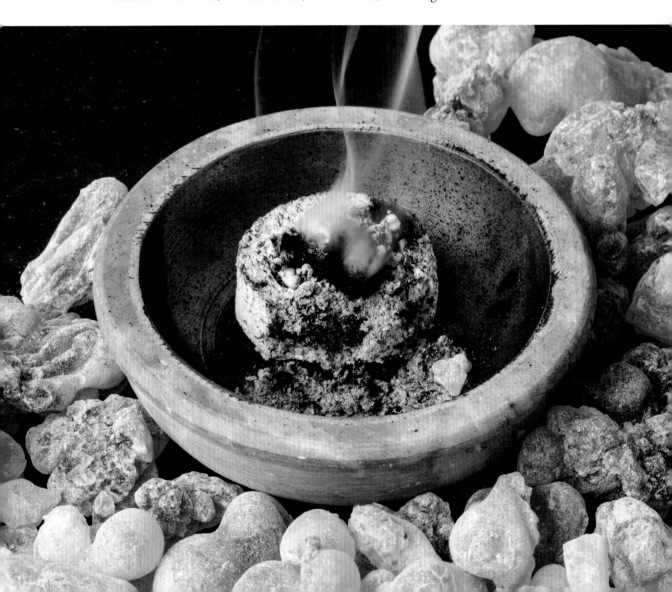

MYRRH

Another gift from the wise men, myrrh is not an herb but a resin extracted from a species of small thorny trees. Myrrh is often used to alleviate the symptoms of nervous system disorders, and researchers have also discovered benefits in the treatment of gastric ulcers, tumors, and parasites. Myrrh gum was used by the ancients to treat infections, toothaches, and various skin conditions.

Associated with purification and cleansings, the scent of myrrh is said to boost the spirit and the soul. Because the aroma is fairly strong, it's often used in conjunction with other herbs or resins, like frankincense or sandalwood. **Myrrh helps you sink into rich and rewarding meditations for introspective purposes, and it is famously used to heal personal sorrow and to connect with the dead in the spirit world.**

USING INCENSE RESINS CEREMONIALLY

When you think of incense, you likely imagine the long, self-burning sticks or perhaps the cone-shaped versions. Resins, however, are the oldest forms of incense, used long before sticks or cones, and they remain a popular way of burning incense for spiritual rituals and ceremonies today. Burning resins takes just a bit more care than quickly putting a lighter to the popular incense sticks or cones, but it is the purest way of using incense that there is. We believe it delivers a more potent, spiritually charged experience when used in ritual or ceremony. In fact, burning incense resin is the most typical way churches, mosques, and temples burn incense all over the world.

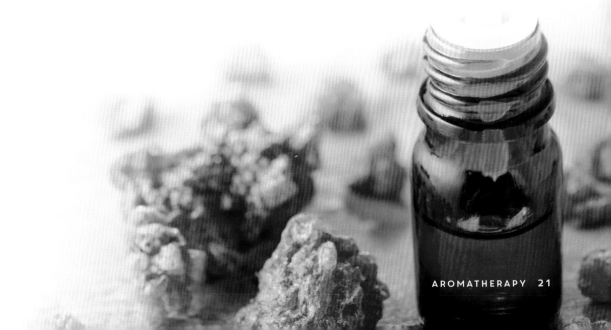

Here's how you can burn incense resins at home for meditation, enjoyment, and ritual.

ITEMS NEEDED:

- Natural ash or sand
- Fire-safe incense holder that can withstand intense heat and temperature change (soapstone, marble, terra-cotta, aluminum, etc.)
- Self-igniting charcoal puck (search for "self-lighting charcoal" on the Internet if you don't know where to buy these locally)
- Metal tongs
- Matches or lighter
- Incense resin (try starting with a frankincense and myrrh mix)

HOW TO BURN INCENSE RESIN:

1. Place about 2 inches of ash or sand in an incense holder, forming a cone shape or mound.

2. Holding the charcoal puck with metal tongs, light the edge until you see tiny sparks.

3. Place the charcoal puck (concave side up) on top of the ash or sand mound, being careful to leave the edges exposed for air to flow around the charcoal.

4. Allow the charcoal to sit for a couple of minutes, until it glows red hot and is covered with gray ash.

5. Sprinkle a small amount of the resin in the indention. About ¼ to ½ teaspoon is enough, as more may smother the charcoal. (Be careful not to touch the charcoal, as it is very hot.)

6. Enjoy the aroma and smoke of the burning incense, feeling free to add more resin as the smoke thins out. The charcoal puck will remain hot for up to an hour, so it's best not to discard it for at least 2 hours to allow proper cooling time. Discard in a fire-safe receptacle.

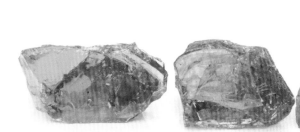
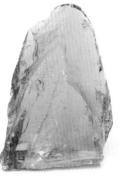

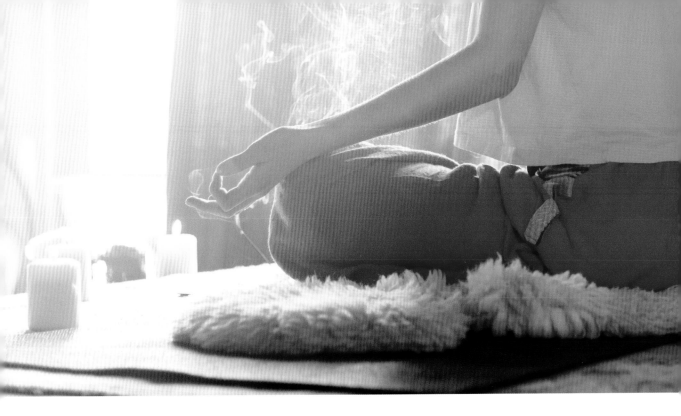

INCENSES AND THEIR USES

TO HELP WITH ...	TRY BURNING ...
Difficulty sleeping	Lavender, rosemary, jasmine, rose
Stress and anxiety	Sandalwood, cherry, pine, vanilla, coconut, benzoin, cypress
Attracting abundance	Jasmine, allspice, bayberry, bergamot, clove, honeysuckle, oakmoss
Meditation	Nag champa, amber, aloe, angelica, anise, gotu kola, lotus, nutmeg
Mental clarity and balance	Patchouli, basil, cardamom, peppermint, sage, violet
Love and romance	Rose, cinnamon, ambergris, carnation, ginger, hibiscus, mastic, mint, musk, ylang-ylang
Courage	Basil, bergamot, cardamom, musk, rose, rose geranium
Protection	African violet, althea, angelica, cedarwood, copal, eucalyptus

CRYSTAL HEALING

"A turquoise given by a loving hand carries with it happiness and good fortune."

—Arabic proverb

What if you knew that beautiful, healing objects were right under your feet? The earth freely offers us crystals, gems, and minerals, which have long been regarded as powerful, living beings for healing and spiritual balance. Mother Earth has always provided all we need to build and to live an optimal, balanced life—and crystals have been one of her most coveted tools for doing so.

Most crystals are minerals formed within the earth as a result of intense heat and pressure. Their atoms and molecules line up in a perfect geometric formation that creates a unique energy signature. Humans also have their own vibrational energy, which varies from person to person and depends on such factors as personality, illness or disease, emotional state, and more. When a healing crystal is brought into a person's energy field, a process of *entrainment* happens. **Entrainment is when your energy field senses the vibrational energy of the crystal and starts to align with it or to vibrate at the same frequency.**

Think this sounds a little "out there"? Nikola Tesla showed how certain forms of energy can alter the vibrational resonance of other forms of energy. *Everything* is vibrational energy, even the most seemingly solid things, and crystals are no different. Because crystals have a fixed structure with a steady vibrational energy, human energy entrains to the crystal's energy, rather than the other way around. It's nature's way of harmonizing discordant vibrations and bringing them into balance.

Our minds, bodies, and spirits can benefit from each crystal's distinct vibrational healing properties and their ability to magnify our own energy. **Crystals are used to facilitate healing; remove energy blockages; enhance meditation; and align body, mind, and spirit.** Various crystals are said to align with different astrological signs, chakras (energy centers in the body), cycles of the moon, and energy frequencies.

How to Choose a Crystal

Crystals come in so many different shapes, sizes, formations, colors, opacities, and lattice structures that it can seem overwhelming to know which one to choose. Surprise: you don't have to! The funny thing about crystals is that they choose *you*. By first tapping into your intuition and declaring your heart-centered intention to receive the perfect crystal for you, all you need to do is walk around a crystal shop or browse online and observe which gems you are most called to. Don't overthink it and don't second guess. Your first impression is typically the right one.

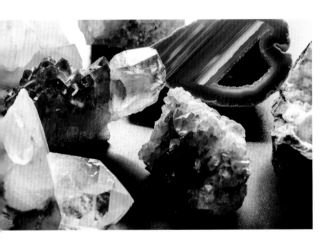

When you sense yourself being drawn to a particular crystal, pick it up (or gaze at it online) and *feel* its energy. What does that crystal evoke within you? Then, and only then, look up what the crystal is used for and its distinct healing benefits. You will most likely discover that the physical and metaphysical properties of the crystal are what you need in your life at that time. And so, that's the crystal for you!

It's important to note that, because crystal healing has grown more popular in the past decade, it is ever more important to shop intentionally from suppliers who source crystals sustainably and with conscious intention to not overharvest these precious gifts from Mother Earth. Crystals from a big-box store? Probably not a good idea, both for the environment and for your energetic resonance. As energy amplifiers, crystals carry the vibration of the entire crystal harvest process, from extraction to your hands, so it matters. When searching for your crystals, ask where they originated and how they were mined.

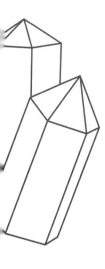

Five Essential Crystals for Maximum Soul Magic

There are thousands and thousands of beautiful and powerful crystals in the world, and that can be overwhelming when searching for your starter crystals. If you're just beginning your crystal collection, these five common crystals will more than cover your bases and help elevate your vibe.

AMETHYST

Ancient civilizations highly valued amethyst and it has long been considered a stone of luxury and protection. Amethyst can be found in all corners of the world, and although this beautiful purple crystal is known for many things, manifestation is at the top of the list.

METAPHYSICAL HEALING PROPERTIES: Connect to your heart's desires and life's purpose with amethyst, and then manifest them in your life! This powerful crystal is associated with the upper chakras, specifically the crown, helping us bring the ethereal realm to the physical plane. This includes bringing our earthly dreams to life.

PHYSICAL HEALING PROPERTIES: The Greek word *amethyst* means "not drunken," so this stone is a good choice for maintaining sobriety. You can also use amethyst to boost the sympathetic nervous system, balance hormones, relieve headaches, ease neck tension, and treat insomnia. Place amethyst under your pillow at night to sleep deeply and wake rested, ready to create and manifest with a purified mind.

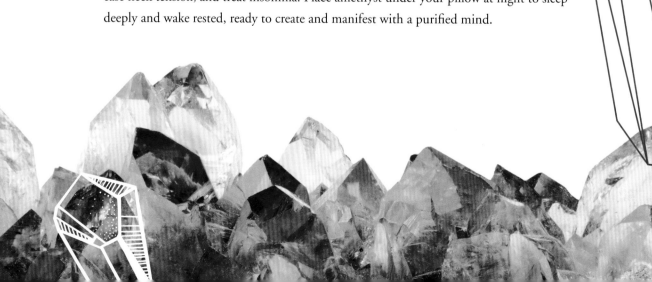

BLACK TOURMALINE

The preferred talisman of protection, black tourmaline is used as a psychic shield to ground your energy and to combat the entry of negative entities into your energy field. Long used by wizards, shamans, witches, and magicians, tourmaline can be found on every continent and is a crystal every energy-sensitive empath needs in their life.

METAPHYSICAL HEALING PROPERTIES: Although tourmaline is black as night, it can be used to ward off negative energies, raise your vibration, and usher you into a brighter light. This stone acts as a sponge for darker energies. It encourages you to remain radiant during dark times, which goodness knows everyone needs!

PHYSICAL HEALING PROPERTIES: Use tourmaline to ease pain in the joints and to assist in realigning the spine. It can also be used to strengthen the immune system, heart, and adrenal glands—easing stress and releasing tension.

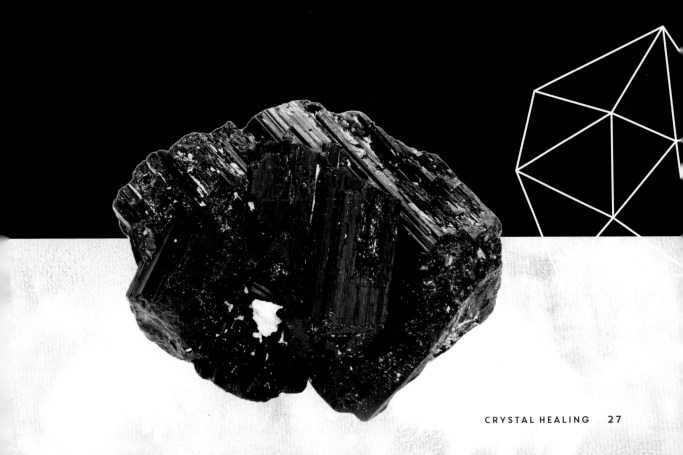

CLEAR QUARTZ

This abundant crystal is a great gift of Mother Earth. Probably the most commonly known crystal, clear quartz is seen as the window of light into the metaphysical world.

METAPHYSICAL HEALING PROPERTIES: Quartz crystal contains the entire color spectrum and can be used to amplify desires, prayers, and manifestations. Meditate with crystal quartz and "program" the crystal with your intentions. You can then wear or carry your crystal with you to raise your vibration and to increase the manifestations of your desires.

PHYSICAL HEALING PROPERTIES: Crystal quartz is a master healer and is thought to stimulate the immune and circulatory systems, increase the flow of qi energy in the body, and open the mind and heart to higher guidance.

"Quartz crystals are the manifestation of the Creator's finest hour of expression."

—*Beverly Criswell,*
Quartz Crystals: A Celestial Point of View

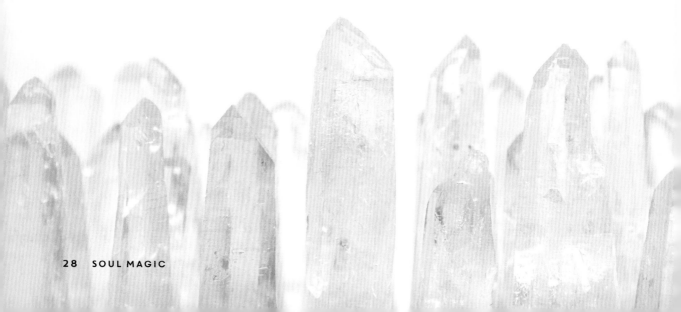

LAPIS LAZULI

This beautiful blue stone has long been associated with royalty and luxury, and its celestial properties assist those in the physical realm with wisdom and good judgment.

METAPHYSICAL HEALING PROPERTIES: Lapis lazuli activates the ethereal upper chakras and empowers the throat chakra for clear communication and ease of expressing one's ideas. This intriguing stone promotes inner observation and truth as it assists in the discovery and representation of the spirit realm.

PHYSICAL HEALING PROPERTIES: Use this powerful stone to support and help heal the throat, larynx, and vocal cords. Due to its strong ties to the brain, it is believed to ease attention deficit disorder (ADD) by helping the mind focus and let go of unnecessary thoughts.

SELENITE

The master crystal, selenite can be used for just about everything, including cleansing other crystals—an important process in crystal healing that we describe below. Selenite is the most abundant crystal in nature and is found in ancient evaporated salt lakes and seas.

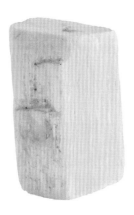

METAPHYSICAL HEALING PROPERTIES: Selenite is a conduit to the highest level of consciousness and all that is infinite—spirit guides, the universe, intuition, and our higher self. It brings the spirit world to Earth and reminds us where we come from, and where we are going after this life.

PHYSICAL HEALING PROPERTIES: Known for its master healing properties, there isn't much that selenite can't be used for. Meditating on a desired outcome for any physical ailment and carrying the stone with you can help to bring great healing and boost inner peace.

How to Work with Crystals

There are many ways you can work with crystals to affect real change in your life. Crystals are an excellent tool to use alone or in conjunction with other healing methods, such as tarot cards (see page 173), meditation (see page 127), and aromatherapy (see page 10). **Crystals are often integrated into feng shui, the Chinese system of object placement to promote the circulation of life force energy, or *chi*. By placing certain crystals in strategic locations based on the feng shui *bagua* (a map or chart of the flow of energy within a home), you can enhance a particular aspect of your life, such as love, abundance, or career.** Many people also wear crystals, usually in jewelry, for the emotional and spiritual qualities they bestow on the wearer. No matter which healing method you choose, an important aspect of working with crystals is knowing how to program them and cleansing them regularly.

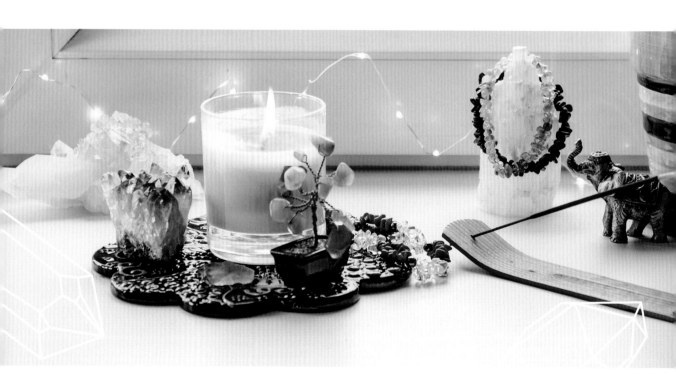

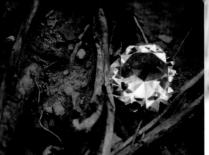
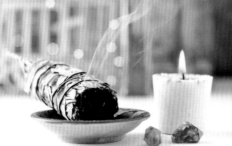
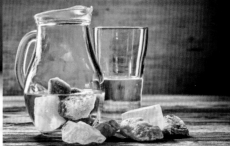

Cleansing Your Crystals

It's important to cleanse your crystals before and after working with them because they can absorb unwanted energy. Cleansing is particularly important if someone else handles your crystals, if you haven't used them in a while, or if you used them for an intense healing session. Here are some ways to cleanse your stones:

BURN: Immerse your crystal in the smoke of a burning sage, palo santo, incense, or any herb that calls to you.

LIGHT: Place your crystal out in the light of the sun for at least four hours, or overnight in the light of the full moon.

SOUND: Using singing bowls or tuning forks can reset the energy of your crystals with the vibration of sound. If you have a singing bowl, place the crystal inside and go to town. With tuning forks, you can just direct the sound to the crystal on a table or other flat surface.

BURY: Crystals are from the Earth and love to go home for a bit. Bury your crystal in the ground and allow it to become recharged with Mother Earth energy.

CRYSTAL MAGIC: Selenite and clear quartz crystals can be used to cleanse the energy of other crystals. Place your crystal in a grid like the ones shown on page 39 and leave overnight. You can buy crystal grids online or make your own.

WASH: Many people recommend using saltwater or spring water to cleanse and "wash" crystals. This is a great way to return your crystal to nature, but please note that some crystals cannot get wet as they will decompose and can become damaged. A quick Google search will give you a list of which crystals cannot be submerged.

Programming a Crystal

It's fascinating to think that quartz crystal is used in many types of modern technology, including sonar, ultrasound, radios, transistors, computer chips, and even digital watches. Why? Because crystals can be programmed and will retain that programming to perform a "task" until programmed otherwise.

Programming your crystals for ritual, manifestation, or healing is a simple and powerful way to integrate your intentions. Crystals retain energy, so when that energy is intentionally and thoughtfully directed at the crystal, your shiny ally will help you create modern-day magic!

FIRST: Cleanse your crystal in one of the ways mentioned on page 31.

NEXT: Hold your crystal in your hands, close your eyes, and take three deep breaths. Reflect on what gives you the most joy, as this will connect you with your highest vibration and open your heart.

NOW: Program your crystal by saying to yourself or aloud, "I ask that the highest vibration of love and light connect with my highest self to clear all unwanted energy or any previous programming. I invite this crystal to hold the intention of (fill in your intention here)."

FINISH: Say thank you three times from your heart and feel the energy envelop your crystal. The more you mean it and really *feel* the gratitude, the better.

Your crystal is now programmed and can be placed in a safe place where you'll see it often in order to remind yourself of your intention. This can be in your bedroom, bathroom, kitchen, desk, or on your altar—the most important thing is to think of a place where it won't be moved or knocked over.

Crystals and the Chakras

Your body is pulsating with energy. Chakras are the energy centers that serve as connection points between the physical body and the spiritual self. A series of seven chakra points run along the spinal column. Each chakra is associated with specific body systems, colors, emotional and spiritual issues, and energetic vibrations. (Again with the energy!) So, crystals are perfectly suited to work with your chakras and balance your energy. **The color of the crystal often aligns with the color associated with each chakra.**

You can place a crystal on the corresponding chakra while meditating. Imagine the healing vibrations of the crystal entering the chakra and aligning the chakra's energy with the crystal's energy (entrainment). You can also do a full chakra balancing with a crystal on each chakra.

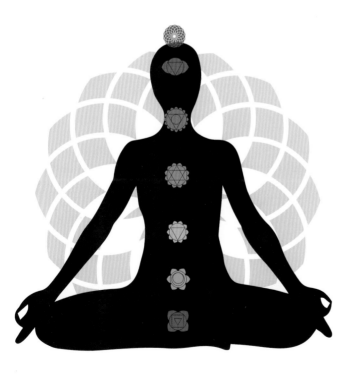

 SAHASRARA

CROWN
Connection of Godness, the Divine Source

 AJNA

THIRD EYE
Wisdom and spiritual awakening

 VISHUDDHA

THROAT
Creativity and communication

 ANAHATA

HEART
Love and kindness

 MANIPURA

SOLAR PLEXUS
Willpower and self-confidence

 SVADHISTHANA

SACRAL
Sexuality and sensuality

 MULADHARA

BASE
Sense of safety and grounding

CHAKRA	LOCATION	COLORS	CRYSTAL PAIRINGS	SPIRITUAL QUALITIES
Root	Base of your spine	Red and black	Garnet, obsidian, ruby	Safety, grounding, protection
Sacral	A few inches below your belly button	Orange and brown	Smoky quartz, carnelian, aragonite	Integrity, identity, control
Solar plexus	Bottom of your sternum	Yellow and gold	Citrine, pyrite, yellow tiger's eye	Self-esteem, courage, maturity
Heart	Center of your chest	Pink and green	Orgonite, rose quartz, emerald	Love, compassion, balance
Throat	Middle of your neck at the throat	Blue and indigo	Blue lace agate, chalcedony, celestite	Truth, communication, self-expression
Third eye	Center of your forehead	Purple and violet	Amethyst, lepidolite, charoite	Intuition, psychic ability, relationship with higher self
Crown	Just above the top of your head	White and clear	Clear quartz, howlite, apophyllite	Ethics, values, connection to Spirit

Crystals for Healing

With so many crystals on Earth, how do you know which ones to use and for what? Here is a quick guide. You'll want to do more research to target your own situation and unique needs.

FINDING LOVE

Amber   Garnet
Moonstone   Rose quartz
Amethyst   Green aventurine
Pink topaz   Ruby

Rose quartz *can be used when seeking love, cultivating self-love, dealing with depression and anxiety, and enhancing fertility.*

ATTRACTING ABUNDANCE

Pyrite   Citrine
Green jade   Green aventurine
Clear quartz Selenite
Emerald

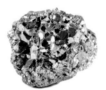

Pyrite, *called "fool's gold," can help bring good fortune your way.*

HEALING FROM TRAUMA

Aventurine   Amazonite
Labradorite   Rhodochrosite
Jade charoite Chrysocolla

OVERCOMING CREATIVE BLOCKS

Carnelian   Citrine
Chrysoprase   Amethyst
Herkimer diamond   Apatite
Tangerine quartz   Bloodstone
Celestite

DEALING WITH ANXIETY AND DEPRESSION

Sodalite   Howlite
Moonstone   Rose quartz
Kyanite   Shungite

ENHANCING FERTILITY

Amber   Aventurine
Rose quartz   Unakite
Sunstone

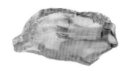

Amber has mystical properties and can be used to enhance fertility.

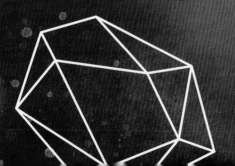

Making a Crystal Elixir

Aside from coffee and Red Bull, can you *drink* energy? Yes, you can—by infusing water with the vibrational frequency of crystals! Simply pour water into a clean glass jar, put it in another container, and surround the outside of the jar with crystals, allowing the crystals to touch the jar. Leave it undisturbed for 24 hours. The vibrational frequency of the stones will transfer to the water. Or, place a water-safe crystal in a glass jar of water and let it soak for 24 hours. Many crystals are not safe to ingest, but clear, rose, and smoky quartz are all safe, as well as amethyst. You can then use the water in numerous ways:

- Drink it.
- Add it to bathwater.
- Put it in a spray bottle and spritz an area with it.
- Add it to nontoxic cleaning products and use it to clean surfaces in your home.
- Add it to shampoo or conditioner and wash your hair with it.

Wearing Crystals

Crystals are beautiful, but that's not the only reason to wear them. Get strategic about where you want to bring healing based on the chakras.

Earrings are associated with your upper chakras, the throat, third eye, and crown. To encourage a healthy energy flow in those areas, wear crystals that align with the colors of these chakras: blue/indigo, purple/violet, or white/clear.

A necklace or pendant can rest on your throat chakra, heart chakra, or solar plexus, depending on the length of the chain. Crystals to choose for these chakras are blue/indigo, pink/green, or yellow/gold.

Crystals worn on *bracelets* are connected to the solar plexus (yellow/gold), sacral chakra (orange/brown), and root chakra (red/black). This is also the place to wear crystals if you wish to bring healing energy to your arms or hands.

Anklets are aligned with the root chakra (red/black) and can help bring healing to the hips, legs, and feet.

And finally, *rings*, aligned with the solar plexus (yellow/gold), sacral chakra (orange/brown), and root chakra (red/black), can be especially powerful. You can direct energy to specific locations depending on which hand and which finger you wear the ring on:

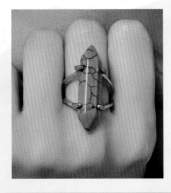

Right hand	analytical mind
Left hand	subconscious mind
Thumbs	self-care
Pointer fingers	desire, ambition
Middle fingers	power
Ring fingers	commitment, love
Pinkies	boundaries, relationships

Crystals and Meditation

Because they amplify energy, crystals are an excellent accompaniment for meditation (see page 127). Choose a stone that aligns with your intention for the meditation, whether that is an intention for clarity, stillness, peace, ease, or something else. Then try these techniques:

- Hold your crystal of choice in your receiving hand (this is your nondominant hand). Use the feeling of the crystal in your hand as a point of focus to still your mind.
- Place the crystal in front of you and gaze at it with a soft focus to center your mind.
- For a movement meditation, such as walking or dancing, place the crystal in a pocket or wear it around your neck. As you focus on your movements, notice how the crystal helps you feel grounded and connected to the earth.
- Try this full-body crystal meditation that helps align each chakra. Lying down, create a crystal grid on your body: above the head on the ground, at the third eye, on the cheekbones and/or chin, throat, heart, solar plexus, sacral, root, and feet. Tap into the energy of each crystal and invite that energy into your energy field.

Sleep with Your Crystals

A profound way to integrate crystal healing into your daily life is to sleep with a programmed crystal (see page 32) under your pillow. Our subconscious mind takes the wheel when we are sleeping, making it the best time to integrate and absorb the intentions placed on our programmed crystal. Take your crystal to bed with you and meditate on your intention before placing it under your pillow and falling asleep. Not all crystals are good bedmates, however, and some can keep you awake. Selenite, howlite, and all quartz stones are safe bets.

Crystal Grids

Don't worry—you don't need any graph paper for this! A crystal
"grid" isn't necessarily a box of intersecting lines (although it can be).
Crystal grids come in many shapes and formats and unite the energies
of a collection of crystals. They are a powerful way to hold your
intention and use geometry to amplify the energy to the universe.

There are many ways to create a crystal grid:

• Print a sacred geometry symbol of your choosing and place cleansed and programmed
  crystals at the intersecting points on the lines.

• Intutively place the crystals in a shape that calls to you.

• Research specific shapes and crystal positions for specific intentions and healing.

With crystal grids, there will always be a center crystal into which all the energy of the
surrounding crystals is directed. It is best if this is a pointed quartz crystal, but any
crystal you feel aligned with will do. The following images show common crystal grids.
You can find these online or make your own.

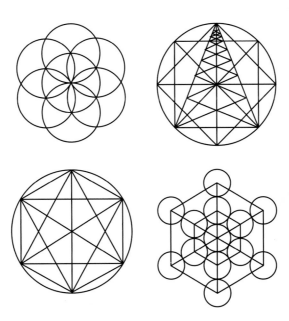

HERBALISM

"Let your foods be your medicines, and your medicines your food."

—*Hippocrates*

Just as the healing power of crystals is beneath our feet, the healing power of plants is easily at hand. Plants are our oldest allies and the most natural healers on this planet. Long before we had scientific proof that certain herbs and plants alleviated specific ailments, we had intuition and magic to show us the way. We simply listened to the plants and recognized that they had a lot to teach us.

Prior to the age of modern medicine, we relied solely on nature for healing. There is much to learn from the creativity, diversity, and resiliency of Mother Nature. To our ancestors, it was everything—and so, through the millennia, they discovered and documented *a lot* about how the plant world can help us. As discussed in the aromatherapy section of this book (page 10), the essences and scents of plants have incredible healing power. Here, we'll explore the use of plants and herbs as natural medicine.

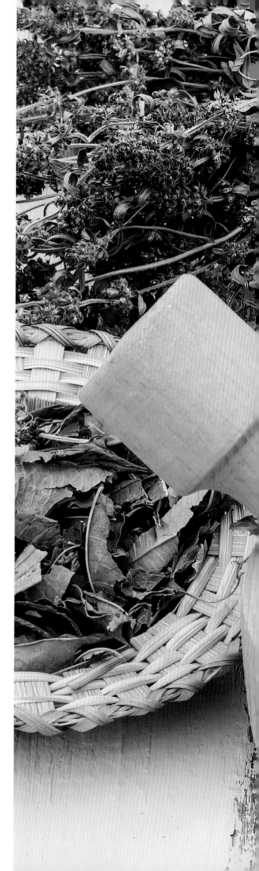

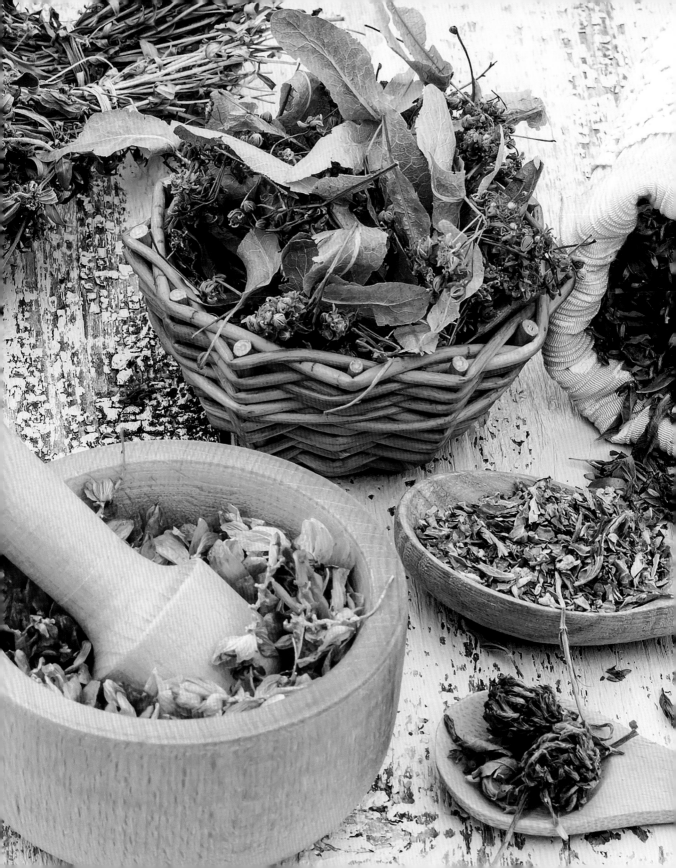

"All plants are our brothers
and sisters. They talk
to us and if we listen,
we can hear them.

—*Arapaho saying*

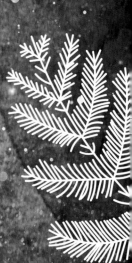

Sometimes referred to as folk medicine or alternative medicine, plant medicine, or herbology—the use of herbs for medicinal purposes and natural healing—is the oldest form of medicine known to humans. Our ancestors listened to the land, watched the animals and what they ate, and made intuitive connections between plants and healing. They learned that plants influence more than just the physical body—plants influence the spiritual body, too. It's no wonder that plants were coveted and used as currency in trade and were transported far and wide with great care. This rich understanding and use of herbs gave rise to Traditional Chinese Medicine as well as the Indian healing system of Ayurveda.

Modern Herbalism

Many of the herbs used in common pharmaceuticals today were used in their basic and rudimentary forms 5,000 years ago to alleviate the same ailments. The astonishing fact that corporate pharmaceutical companies still go to rainforests, deserts, and mountain ranges for ingredients proves that nature has indeed not lost its potency, and never will. But, more often than not, we don't need Big Pharma to treat our ailments. We have the power to grow our own herbs, create custom remedies, and reconnect with the age-old practice of herbalism.

Ancestral Truths

As far back as 5,000 years ago in ancient Mesopotamia, clay tablets were used to keep track of various herbs and their specific uses. These tablets are the oldest written record we have about the use of plants as medicine.

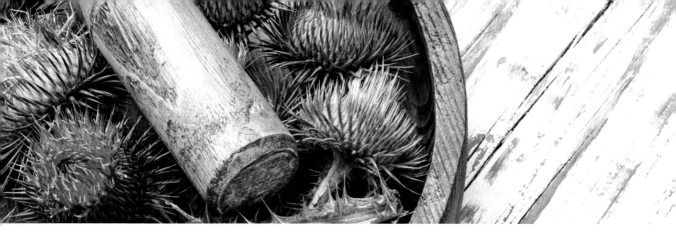

Everyday Herbs for Self-Healing

It's time to begin regaining our power over our own health and
wellness. Here are five powerful herbs that can be found right in your
kitchen or local apothecary and a few of their medicinal benefits
and uses, although there are thousands more herbs to explore.

OREGANO: Originating from Greece, this potent herb is a natural infection fighter. It
is commonly used to treat gingivitis, toenail fungus, bronchitis, yeast infections, urinary
tract infections, bacterial vaginosis, ringworm, athlete's foot, sinus infections, and more.
Oregano oil (not to be confused with the essential oil) can be ingested orally in capsule
or liquid form. However, do not place oregano oil directly on the skin, as it will burn.

ROSEMARY: Native to the Mediterranean region, rosemary is one of the most
versatile herbs, with a wide array of healing benefits. It stimulates hair growth, improves
memory and brain function, reduces liver damage, lowers stress, balances hormones,
prevents blood clots, and has anti-inflammatory, antibacterial, and antimicrobial
properties. You can make rosemary tea, add rosemary to recipes, use the essential oil,
infuse water with the herb, or get creative and try something new!

MILK THISTLE: Used for more than 2,000 years, milk thistle was revered by the
ancient Greeks for its healing properties. Milk thistle has antioxidant, antiviral, and anti-
inflammatory properties. It is used to detoxify the liver, draw out toxins from the body

that can cause cancer, lower cholesterol levels, and more. Try taking milk thistle on an empty stomach, 20 minutes before a meal, for best results.

GARLIC: Many ancient civilizations the world over have used garlic as a remedy. Garlic has been linked to the prevention of the four leading causes of death: heart disease, cancer, infection, and stroke. It can be used to treat the common cold, boost the immune system, lower blood pressure, help prevent heart disease and cancer, reverse hair loss, improve symptoms of dementia, and treat diabetes. Take raw garlic, or garlic supplements, daily or at the first sign of a cold.

LEMON BALM: Our ancestors cultivated lemon balm for medicinal use and regarded it as an elixir of long life when taken daily. Lemon balm improves digestion and the expulsion of bile from the gallbladder, reduces stress and anxiety, helps with insomnia, decreases free radicals, and regulates the thyroid. It can be taken in tea or tincture form, and the essential oil can be used topically.

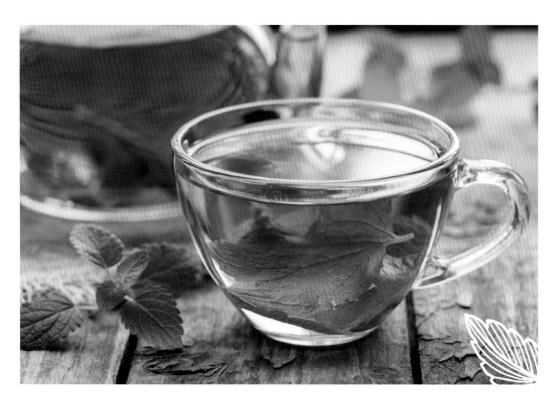

Magical Herbs 101

Ready to take it up a notch and experiment with the magical properties of plants? Here are a few suggestions to add some soul magic to your life.

MUGWORT: Mugwort has a very long history. It has been used as a medicine, for spiritual purposes (including astral travel and divination), in acupuncture treatments, and even as an ingredient in beer! Try using mugwort incense to cleanse your divination objects, such as tarot cards, crystals, and pendulums.

YARROW: Achilles, the Greek hero whom yarrow is named after, is said to have used yarrow on the battlefield to heal wounds. It is also used to heal emotional wounds. Add dried yarrow to a sachet and place it near your bed to help ward off nightmares and resolve trauma.

ROSE PETALS: Roses are essential for every botanical arsenal. It may not be a surprise that they are used for love spells, to express appreciation and sympathy, and to support the emotional heart. Drink a cup of rosebud tea before going to bed to help ease and calm your mind and induce prophetic dreams.

RUE: Early physicians considered rue an extraordinary defender against plague. As a great protector, rue was also used to ward off evil spirits and curses and to safeguard the home. Try planting rue in a little vessel near your front door to prevent negative energy from entering your home. Be cautious if you have pets or children, though, as rue can be poisonous in large doses.

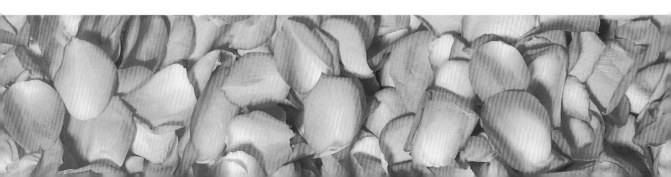

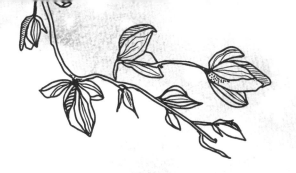

Tip for a Magical Sleep

Mugwort is a potent herbal ally and a reliable
lucid dream enhancer to facilitate dream recall! One
powerful way to work with mugwort is to make a dream
pillow. It is very easy and inexpensive to make. First, purchase dried
mugwort and fill a small cotton drawstring bag (both can be found
at health food stores, apothecaries, or online shops, such as Mountain
Rose Herbs). You can add aromatic herbs, such as mint, lavender, and
chamomile, to the mix as well. Place the satchel under your pillow or on your
nightstand. Set an intention for your dreams before bed—such as assistance
revealing an answer to a question you may have or connecting with a
spirit guide. Drift off to sleep and let your magic pillow do its thing!
Be sure to keep a dream journal next to your bed to write down all
that you remember, or record a voice note in your phone.

Adaptogens

Adaptogens literally help us adapt! These herbs, roots, and mushrooms can help combat stress, anxiety, adrenal fatigue, insomnia, hormonal imbalances, mental fogginess, fatigue, and so much more. Adaptogens are available in powder and capsule form. Some of our favorite adaptogens that have tremendous healing benefits include:

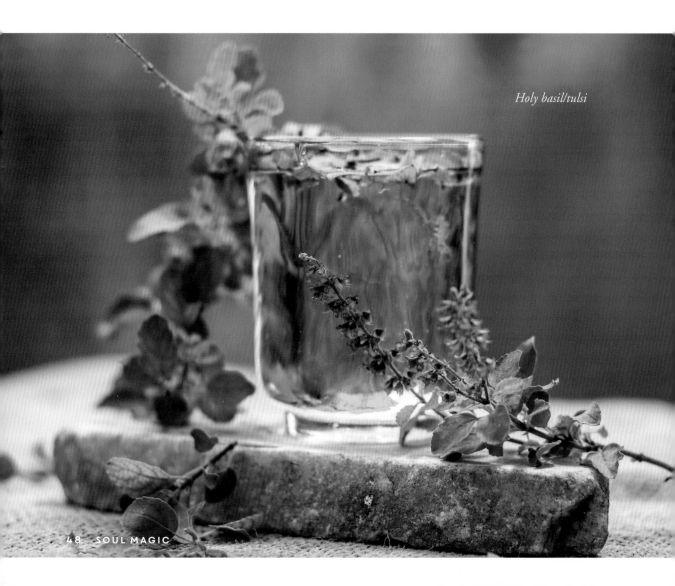

Holy basil/tulsi

Chaga mushrooms	lower cholesterol, prevent and fight cancer, support the immune system, fight inflammation
Turkey tail mushrooms	powerful antioxidant, support the immune system, balance gut bacteria
Lion's mane mushrooms	protect against aging and dementia, reduce anxiety and depression, help repair nerve damage
Shiitake mushrooms	support the immune system, lower blood cholesterol levels, ease syptoms of eczema, treat colds and flu
Cordycep mushrooms	support the immune system, enhance athletic performance, promote longevity, support liver, kidney, and sexual health
Reishi mushrooms	reduce stress, improve sleep, lessen fatigue, lower high blood pressure and cholesterol, support the immune system
Ashwagandha	help fight depression, boost fertility and testosterone in men, boost brain function, reduce anxiety
Rhodiola	reduce stress, fight fatigue, balance hormones, help fight depression, improve brain function, control diabetes, potential anticancer properties
Holy basil/tulsi	reduce stress and anxiety, fight inflammation, antioxidant, arthritis and fibromyalgia support
Maca	gain muscle and increase strength, boost energy, balance hormones, treat symptoms of menopause, improve fertility and sexual potency
Ginseng	powerful antioxidant, reduce inflammation, boost brain function, improve erectile dysfunction, boost energy, lower blood sugar, aphrodisiac
Turmeric	prevent heart disease, fight inflammation, reduce pain, antioxidant, help fight depression, arthritis support

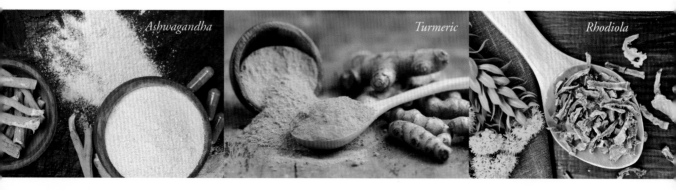

Ashwagandha *Turmeric* *Rhodiola*

Herbalism vs. Plant Medicine

Recently, "plant medicine" has seen a wave of popularity in the West as more and more people are searching for alternative ways of healing. By returning to the plants, and to trusted shamans who have used them for centuries as medicine, we can heal physically as well as spiritually, attaining deeper meaning in our lives.

Plant medicine most commonly refers to ingesting a plant that will alter your state of consciousness. Whether the plant is cannabis or ayahuasca, cacao or psilocybin, the plants offer a different realm of healing altogether. While herbalism surely is plant medicine at its core, what we are talking about when we say "plant medicine" is medicine for the soul. Herbalism, on the other hand, is more focused on relieving the symptoms and root causes of physical and emotional ailments.

Many people are seeking out plant medicine in order to transcend reality, obtain psychedelic effects, and connect with the source of all. Many people contend that plant medicine serves to reconnect us to ourselves and our hearts through the power of nature, and to remind us that it is possible to heal on a deep emotional and spiritual level and thrive in the face of life's challenges and traumas.

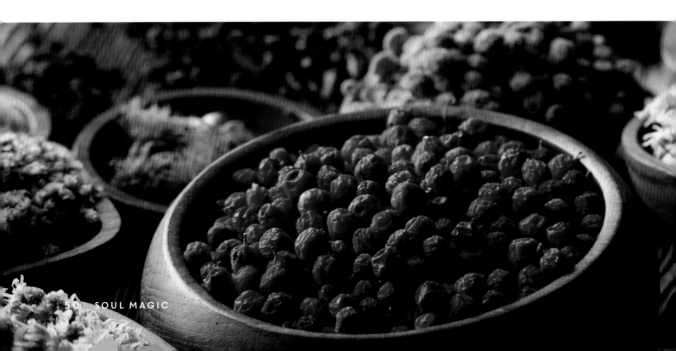

While plant medicine is a core practice of many indigenous tribes and cultures, mainstream society has largely been against plant medicine and its psychedelic properties, with most psychedelic plants classified as Schedule I drugs. However, science is now proving the medicinal benefits of cannabis, psilocybin, cacao, peyote, and other plant medicines. Journeying within and removing oneself from everyday reality with the help of plant allies has been shown to be effective in reducing anxiety and depression, and even PTSD.

The Multidisciplinary Association of Psychedelic Studies (MAPS) is a nonprofit organization working to change U.S. laws on certain drugs, creating a safe way in which we can heal from trauma and mental disease via plant medicine. MAPS develops medical, legal, and cultural contexts for people to benefit from the careful uses of psychedelics and marijuana. This doesn't mean you should hit up that rave happening in the warehouse downtown and buy a mushroom from a stranger, but the more open we are to the healing benefits of mind-altering substances received in safe ceremonial spaces from trusted shamans and spiritual teachers, the more open we will be to our healing and spiritual advancement as a society. The focus is on microdosing and taking a small, controlled amount in a safe environment to heal on a deep emotional and spiritual level.

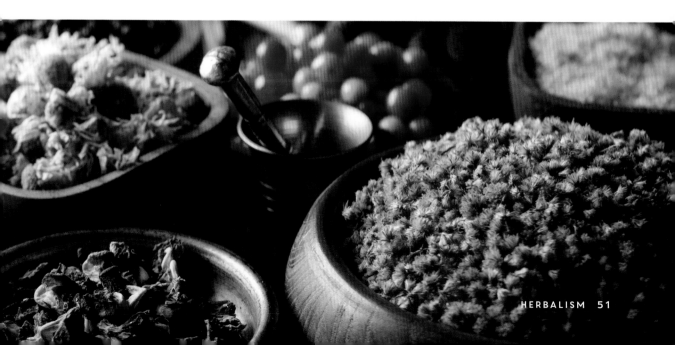

How Does Plant Medicine Work?

———— • ————

Herbs and plants can bring the body back into harmony on a physiological and spiritual level. When certain plants are ingested, they make their way through the body, restoring ease and harmony where there is dis-ease and dis-harmony. We are part of nature—one with nature—and it is nature that can help us heal and recalibrate to our natural state of well-being. We are born to heal, and our plant allies are here to assist us on that journey back to homeostasis.

> "Unlike pharmaceutical drugs, which simply alleviate or numb symptoms of disease, the plants bring the body back into alignment. They cure root causes and conditions. And they do it in the most mysterious of ways."
>
> —*Jane Mayer*

As we go through life, we all are met with multiple challenges—which is why the Buddha made the presence of suffering his First Noble Truth. If you are a human, you will experience pain at some point, or more likely at many points. Some of these challenges will be crippling, some sticky, and some just annoying. **However difficult the challenges we face, the key to addressing them head-on is found in the subconscious mind**. When our pain lodges in the subconscious mind and creates negative patterns, they become blocks in consciousness and can be extremely difficult to transcend. These blocks can and do induce behaviors like addiction, personality disorders, mental health issues, psychological imbalances, and physical manifestations of disease.

Plant medicines help us access these blocks objectively, evaluate them directly, and face the fear that is keeping them alive. Once fear is acknowledged, it loses its power immediately. In the face of plant medicines that bring our subconscious patterns to light, fear doesn't stand a chance. We are botanically supported to confront the issue that is blocking the ease and flow of our consciousness and innate energy. However, plant medicines are *not* a quick fix. It is difficult and vulnerable work to journey with plant medicines, so they should never be used with a casual mentality or haphazardly.

The key with plant medicines is *willingness*. When we are in a state of disease, whether mental, emotional, or physical, operating on fear and living within self-created blocks, the ego thrives. It loves this garden of distress. The ego will do anything to protect this constant fight-or-flight mode because that is when it's in control. The minute the ego loosens control and the heart/soul takes over is the minute that we are free from the confines of fear.

When the heart and soul regain control and lovingly guide us to and through our egoic blocks, we experience what is referred to as "spontaneous healing." This type of healing can happen after just one or two ceremonies sitting with plant medicine, and it has been known to alleviate ailments that range from crippling anxiety to cancer. There are many stories of spontaneous healing from various types of plant medicines, and the fact that people are flocking to ancient jungles, traditional healers, and cultures that revere nature and work *with* it is a testament to our search for connection to something greater than what our society currently provides.

Some plant medicines, such as cannabis and cacao, are lightweights compared to the work that master plants like ayahuasca, peyote, and psilocybin bring forward. The negative stigma that plant medicines—particularly hallucinogens—carry makes them largely illegal globally. This reflects our ego's resistance to them. Plant medicine can remind us of our own power and of our intrinsic connection to nature.

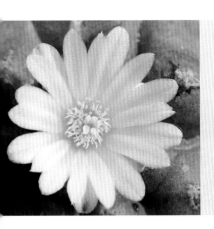

I like to remind others that using plants for healing comes with responsibility. We're supposed to leave some grandmother and grandfather plants to carry on their lineage, not pick every last stem. And we're meant to ask the plants for their permission to be picked.

—*Shannon,* MASTER HERBALIST

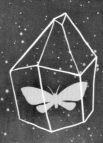

PART 2

PRACTICAL MAGIC

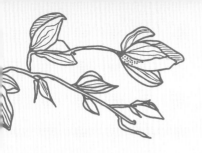

—— ••• ——

You might think the words *practical* and *magic* clash with each other, but the truth is that magic loves to be used in practical ways! This doesn't mean, however, that magic seeks to be confined. The opposite is true: magic is innately creative. The practical use of magic means integrating creativity and structure in a way that brings great joy and abundance into our lives from our infinite source of energy.

We've all heard of manifestation and casting spells. These are perfect examples of using the art and creativity of magic for practical means to help us connect to the divine and humanize its power. Today we are more equipped than ever with practical means of using ancient magic in our everyday lives. When we look back in time, we can begin to understand that we have truly never been *without* this knowledge, and in remembering our ancient roots, we can realize our modern potential.

From manifesting our deepest soul-inspired desires, to quieting the relentless chatter of the mind through a sanctified day of rest, to deciphering the meaning in numbers to plan for our best future, we are divinely supported in wielding practical magic in the daily world. Going far beyond the notion of "abracadabra," practical magic is truly everywhere.

—— ••• ——

MANIFESTATION

"Whatever we plant in our subconscious mind
and nourish with repetition and emotion
will one day become a reality."

—*Earl Nightingale*

The Buddha said, "What you think, you become. What you feel, you attract. What you imagine, you create." This, in essence, is the art of manifestation.

Although the movie *The Secret* made manifestation a popular practice today, the famous ancient sage Hermes Trismegistus, known as the "Master of Masters" in ancient Egypt and Greece, taught all we need to know about the secrets of manifestation long ago. In the ancient Emerald Tablet, Hermes outlined seven principles that the universe—and everything in it, including us—runs on. In order to be able to manifest our ideal life, we must learn to align with these spiritual, natural laws rather than operate from a mere egotistical "give me what I want," flick-of-the-wand mentality. Our egos have been fed to think the universe is here to align with our will, but **the truth is that *we are meant to align with the higher will of universal intelligence through conscious co-creation.***

Nothing happens by chance. That's because we live in a law-based world. There are specific, undeniable laws of the universe that work in synergy to manifest external realities. These laws are always at work, whether we are aware of them or not. However, when we learn to work *with* these laws, that's when we can create our best, most abundant lives.

"Chance is but a name for law not recognized."

—*The Kybalion*

To illustrate this, think about electricity. Many people do not know *how* electricity works on a technical level, yet a lamp still works in their home if they plug it in. If they don't plug it in, electricity goes on "working" just the same, but it won't provide the benefits of its light.

The same goes for the laws of life. If we want to manifest an abundant, limitless life of true freedom, we need to begin by understanding and trusting in these universal laws. All it takes is the knowledge of *how* to plug in.

The Roles of the Conscious and Subconscious Minds

We can't talk about successful manifestation until we address the roles of the two levels of our mind: the conscious and the subconscious.

Our conscious mind is the reasoning mind, and it makes all our daily decisions. It is referred to as the "objective mind" because it deals with the external world and its objects. The conscious mind obtains knowledge through the five senses via observance and experience. Its main function is analysis and reason.

Our subconscious, or subjective, mind, on the other hand, perceives by intuition, completely independent of the five senses. It cannot argue or reason like the conscious mind, so what is suggested to it over and over becomes its truth and operating system. In other words: what you think about all day, you become. Words are spells, even when they are only spoken silently in the mind as thoughts.

"Every thought we think is creating our future."
—*Louise Hay*

Science says that by the age of seven, our subconscious patterns are set in place and will play out for the rest of our lives unless consciously reconditioned. And that's exactly what true manifestation calls for: a reconditioning of our subconscious thoughts and behaviors. Learning the natural laws of the universe—of which manifestation, or attraction, is one—and rewiring our brains around them requires subconscious overhaul and nothing less. In other words, if we program our subconscious with the wrong thoughts, it will accept them as true, and these inaccurate beliefs will drive our behavior and our experiences. Such erroneous beliefs that get programmed into our subconsious are things like: "I am not worthy," "I don't deserve good things," "I am a flawed person," "I must be perfect in order for good things to happen," "Bad things always happen to me," and so on. As the storehouse of memory, the subconscious mind is where the work of manifestation really happens.

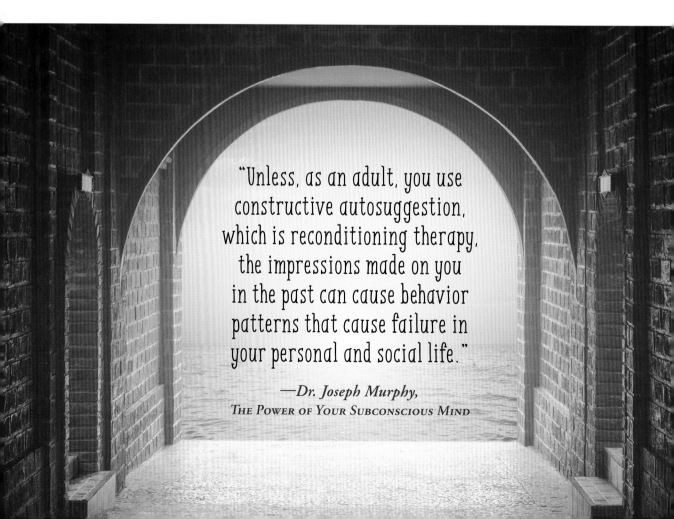

"Unless, as an adult, you use constructive autosuggestion, which is reconditioning therapy, the impressions made on you in the past can cause behavior patterns that cause failure in your personal and social life."

—*Dr. Joseph Murphy,*
THE POWER OF YOUR SUBCONSCIOUS MIND

The Seven Principles of Manifestation

The Emerald Tablet is the foundational text on the power of mental transmutation, or mental alchemy. When you think of the word *alchemy*, your mind probably conjures ideas of turning a base metal like lead into gold, but to the ancient mystics, alchemy was more about the transmutations of the *mind*. To "transmute" means to change in form, nature, or substance; therefore, mental alchemy refers to changing the form of our thoughts and subsequent emotions from negative and destructive to positive and constructive.

Hermes' teachings—called the Hermetic teachings—tell us that there are seven sacred principles that govern our universe and fuel our ability to change the world around us solely with the power of our minds. We discuss the first three here in detail, as they most directly apply to manifestation, but we encourage you to research the seven in more depth for the highest possible understanding.

THE SEVEN HERMETIC PRINCIPLES

1. The Principle of Mentalism: *The All is mind; the universe is mental*

2. The Principle of Correspondence: *As above, so below. As below, so without; as without, so within*

3. The Principle of Vibration: *Nothing rests; everything moves; everything vibrates*

4. The Principle of Polarity: *Everything is dual; everything has poles*

5. The Principle of Rhythm: *Everything flows, out and in; everything has its tides*

6. The Principle of Cause and Effect: *Everything has its cause; everything has its effect*

7. The Principle of Gender: *Gender is in everything; everything has its masculine and feminine principles*

"The principles of truth are seven; he who knows these, understandingly, possesses the magic key before whose touch all the doors of the temple fly open."

—*The Kybalion*

The Principle of Mentalism

You likely have heard the New Age maxim "Thoughts become things."
Well, there is nothing "new" about this buzz phrase. That our thoughts,
feelings, and beliefs bear their own fruit, like seeds sown in the soil, is
a truth known since the furthest reaches of human time, and is told by
the first Hermetic principle, the principle of mentalism. The principle
of mentalism states: "The All is mind; the universe is mental."

The universe itself is made up of mind, and all of creation exists in that universal,
intelligent mind. All phenomena, including all matter and energy, are thoughts in the
mind of God (or Source, Spirit, Higher Power—insert your word of choice here!).

What does this mean for you? It means we are all made from, and part of, the divine,
an intelligent source of energy that creates and permeates *all* of life. And because we are
a small part of the greater whole, we share its characteristics—most importantly, the
ability to create our outer realities with the power of our inner mindsets. In other words,
perception is reality; things are how you think they are. Or, as American essayist Ralph
Waldo Emerson put it, "Man is what he thinks about all day long."

It's important to know that historically, the idea that everything is made up of mind,
or thought—that we are powerful godlike creatures—would have been considered a
radical, often blasphemous concept to the masses. So, this sacred knowledge was hidden
behind "mystery traditions" spearheaded by wise sages and mystics.

This ancient insight, if absorbed and embodied, means that we are powerful enough
to create our own lives exactly as we want them by our internal worlds—our thoughts,
beliefs, and feelings. We might never be able to understand the complete workings of
the intelligent universe fully as humans, but that has very little to do with our ability to
connect with, and benefit from, that source of power. The goal is to understand how this
universal energy works so we can work *with* it to manifest our highest vibrational, most
authentic life. Fully understanding this first principle is vital to successfully executing the
rest of them, and to manifesting effectively.

The Principle of Correspondence

You've probably heard the phrase, "It's all in your head!" And the principle of correspondence shows us that there literally is nothing truer than that. The principle of correspondence states: "As above, so below; as below, so above. As within, so without; as without, so within." This means that we operate in the mirror image in which the greater universe operates. Therefore, building off the first principle, if the universe is mind and creates its reality via thoughts, so do we! Since we are a microcosm of the macrocosm, we'll get clues about how we can take an active role in creating the life of our dreams by observing how the universe creates.

The world outside of you—your current external reality—reflects the world inside of you, that is, your innermost dominant thoughts. Are your thoughts fear based or faith based? Envious or loving? Confident or worrisome? It turns out, it matters *a lot*! The major lesson this principle teaches is that if you don't like your external life circumstances, the place to fix that isn't externally, but internally. This is valuable insight when we consider that most of us default to trying to change things on an external level. But it's when we tend to our inner world first that our external world really begins to shift.

If you're living an inner life of disease, turmoil, self-hate, or toxicity, that is eventually going to manifest in your exterior life in different challenging ways, such as financial difficulty, bad relationships, illness, or depression. If your interior life is focused on positivity, self-empowerment, and self-love, then you're in alignment to manifest a life of grace and ease, full of abundance, purpose, and meaningful relationships.

The principle of correspondence teaches that in order to change your outer life for the better, the change must first start on the inside, with your core beliefs, visualizations, and self-talk. This idea is the basis for the law of attraction and manifestation.

The Principle of Vibration

When we learn to focus the mind and amplify our own vibration, we gain more power to make our dreams come true. We know that everything is energy. And that means that everything is constantly in motion. The principle of vibration states: "Nothing rests; everything moves; everything vibrates."

There are poles of vibration, with high-vibration spirit at one end of the pole and low-vibration, extremely dense forms of matter at the other end. Between the two poles are millions upon millions of different rates of vibration. We are able to slide along higher on the scale toward higher vibration as we practice intention or focusing the mind. When our vibrations continually increase from matter toward spirit, our manifestations become more spiritually inclined as well.

How can we use the principle of vibration to manifest our dreams? When we consciously choose to alter our mood from sad to happy, from angry to forgiving, from despondent to inspired, we are actively amplifying our vibration. Therefore, when we visualize what we want to create, it is key that we feel the happiness as if it's taking place *at this moment*. This is referred to as "living as if." The subconscious can't distinguish between what is actually happening in the outer world and what is being visualized in the inner world. When we experience joyful emotions through visualization, our subconscious reads that as if it were happening in that moment. This amplifies our vibration, and nothing helps manifest more quickly than a heightened, spiritward vibration.

Try sitting in a short meditation, around five minutes, and visualize the life you wish to create, down to the finest details. See it so clearly that you *feel* the happiness that comes with that kind of life. Athletes are trained to do this, and they visualize each play of the game and its ending in a positive way with them winning.

Embodying the Hermetic Principles

The very best thing we can do for the betterment of the world is to make the most of ourselves, and the three ancient Hermetic principles empower us to do just that. The process of manifestation all boils down to understanding and implementing techniques in accordance with the natural laws of the universe that allow us to unify the desires of the conscious and subconscious mind. Believe that you not only have the power to manifest, but that the universe is also doing the work to co-create the life of your dreams. It's a team effort!

Manifestation is merely the ability to shape our reality through mastery of the self, dictated by the natural laws of universal intelligence.

However, universal intelligence is always about manifesting for the greater good. It is not solely about an individual's wants and needs. We will never get what we want if it is out of alignment with the greater "will" of universal intelligence. To truly manifest, we have to yield to the will of the highest good of all concerned and believe—with every ounce of faith inside of us—that the good that's meant for us is already here and that we are deserving and prepared to receive it.

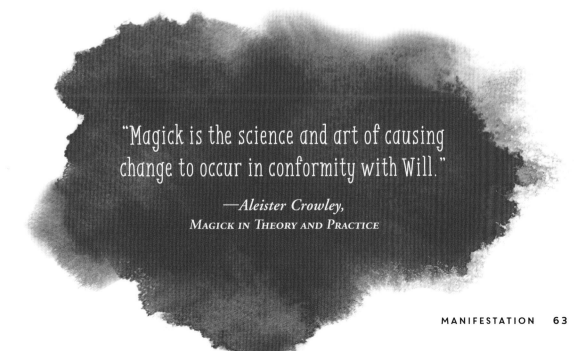

"Magick is the science and art of causing change to occur in conformity with Will."

—*Aleister Crowley,*
Magick in Theory and Practice

Learn the Formula of Manifestation

———— • ————

With clarity at the forefront and gratitude bringing up the rear,
there is a proven formula with ancient roots that will help you call
things into your life that you are ready to graciously receive.

The first step is to decide what you truly desire to bring into reality, but you need to make sure that it is in alignment with the highest will of all concerned, the highest will of spirit. You may want a million-dollar beach house in California, but the highest will might be for you to have a country ranch in New Mexico because that's where your work will help the most people. If your wish is not in alignment with the greater good or with the larger plan, that type of manifestation will not work. Sometimes being less specific helps. If you want to manifest that a positive living situation comes your way—try letting go of deciding where or what it must be or when it must happen. This is non-attachment, and it's a manifestation power play. The odds are you'll get something even better than you could have imagined.

The truth of manifestation is that you are surrendering to the greater intelligence because, ultimately, *we don't really know what's best for us and everyone around us*! Spirit often has a different, better plan for us, and that may not involve what we think we want. It may involve something even better than we could imagine! Not getting what you want, or what you *think* you want, is the universe's way of helping you dodge a

An Attitude of Gratitude

Adopting an attitude of gratitude is the greatest spiritual tool you could ever develop, and it is absolutely vital in manifesting your highest vibration in life. Say "thank you" to whatever divine source you have faith in and really feel the gratitude emanating from your heart. Say thank you for your blessings and your challenges, because they both help you grow on a spiritual level. Tune in to the feeling of receiving your desires and give pure thanks to the universe and to yourself for bringing this into your reality.

> When I really got into manifestation, I visualized my happiest life every day, and sometimes felt so joyful I thought I was living in a daydream. Things started to shift. Within a few months, I met my girlfriend, who is now my wife, and was recruited by a local business that I admired and was able to create my dream job there. When I look back to just a few years ago, I can't believe how much my life has evolved!
>
> —*Chris, 32*

bullet, guiding you to what is best and in most alignment for your highest self. Rejection is simply cosmic redirection! You can ensure that you are in alignment by simply stating your aligned intention: "I am manifesting [enter desire here] OR something better for the highest will of all concerned. Thank you."

Once you're clear on that and in alignment with the higher will, visualize what you want to create, down to the littlest details, *as if it's already happening*, feeling the emotions you would feel when that person/place/thing comes into your life. End your manifestation with a sincere "THANK YOU"—or three!

Then, surrender.

That's all. Don't dwell or try to micromanage the details of *how*. Release any expectations of specific outcomes and just trust that the universe has your back. From there, things will fall into place as they should. Hold the visualization and feelings of the result of what you desire in your mind as much as you can throughout every day, but don't stress about *how* it will happen. Just visualize, feel, and be grateful as much as possible. Have faith that what's yours is yours and being delivered *right now*!

SABBATH

"The Sunday is the core of our civilization, dedicated to thought and reverence. It invites to the noblest solitude and to the noblest society."

—*Ralph Waldo Emerson*

In our hyperactive, go-go-go, tech-crazed society, the idea of taking a few hours, let alone one entire day, to rest and unplug from our modern grind is a near impossibility. With seemingly never-ending to-do lists and taking work home with us becoming the norm, the lines between work and rest have become virtually nonexistent. Especially in the current Western world, taking breaks from our work is viewed as a weakness, which is unfortunate because there is nothing further from the truth. In actuality, rest is vital to our productivity and profundity.

Many of us are overarchingly obsessed with longing for the past and/or anxiety for the future. The present, however, is voraciously consumed and blindly neglected. It's no secret, then, that learning to live in the moment is a key spiritual goal. The ancient practice of Sabbath is a day dedicated to just that: the present moment. Sabbath means to unplug from what is ultimately valueless on a spiritual level by dedicating one day per week to ensuring there is nothing competing with our highest self. We commit, simply and profoundly, to rest each moment, without any "valueless" distractions—no emails to respond to, no cell phones to answer, and no tasks, big or small, that demand to be finished. Ultimately, Sabbath is a day to revel in the things that truly matter on a larger, more inspired level.

"He who cannot rest, cannot work."

—*Harry Emerson Fosdick*, Riverside Sermons

"The faster you run and accomplish a lot of useless things, the more you are dead."

—*Brenda Ueland,*
IF YOU WANT TO WRITE

Sabbath often gets a bad reputation as a day full of tedious spiritual worship, dogmatic rule-following, and serious churchgoing, but that is a misinterpretation. Before you begin to blow off the idea of Sabbath as "no fun," consider these words from Thomas Nelson, author of *Sabbath: The Ancient Practices*: "Sabbath is the holy time where we feast, play, dance, have sex, sing, pray, laugh, tell stories, read, paint, walk, and watch creation in its fullness." Yes, please!

The great secret of the Sabbath is that it is meant to be a day full of *playfulness and delight*, not piety, and not lazily sleeping all day either. If we start to think of Sabbath as a one-day-per-week oasis of calm amid an often chaotic, stormy life, it becomes clear how beneficial a holy day like this is to all of us. The word *holy* simply means to set aside, to not get lost in the sea of everything else. When we strip the religion away, Sabbath simply means to keep one day a week special and sacred, refusing to participate in the mundane. It is part of life's blueprint for a joyful, meaningful existence. Permission is granted for you to make this day, whichever day it falls on, completely yours and customized. Do what your soul wants, needs, and craves!

Rest: It's a Command!

The word *Sabbath* is derived from the Hebrew word for "rest" and literally means "to rest from labor." Unlike many of the self-care modalities in this book, an official day of rest is not an idea seen cross-culturally in ancient times; instead, it is directly derived from the ancient Israelites. Jewish people refer to the Sabbath as the "queen," and that alone should tell you how important a day of sacred rest is.

Nobody should be doing any mundane work on the seventh day of the week, after toiling tirelessly in the tepid waters of the rat race the previous six. Even if these "tepid" waters fill you with joy, passion, and fulfillment because you love your job, you still need to rest to stay sane and grounded in your ultimate spiritual reality.

The ebb and flow of work and rest, expansion and contraction, make up the very fabric of the universe. Rest doesn't merely mean putting down your daily work task, either; the true rest that Sabbath calls for means taking oneself out of the ordinary, out of the routine, out of the mundane. This intentional weekly retreat gives us the opportunity to connect with our spirit and restore our soul—and that is the entire point of investing in a day of rest.

Which Day Is the Sabbath?

Historically, there has always been contentious discussion of which day is the seventh day, exactly. Originally, Sabbath was from Friday evening through Saturday evening. Early Christians celebrated Sabbath on Saturday, but it was switched to Sunday when Christianity moved to Rome. Muslims, who were influenced by both Jews and Christians, chose to keep the day of rest on Friday.

To the modern mystic looking to grow his/her soul, however, the exact day of the week really has little meaning. The important thing is that one day per week be devoted to unplugging from the ever-growing stresses of the modern age and instead resting in whatever brings you joy. Rest and joy *matter* and are indeed the two vital pillars of self-healing and restoration.

Human Being or Human Doing?

Western culture values busyness, speed, and productivity, yet we envy those whose leisure time is abundant. Bragging about how busy we are is practically a national sport, a pillar of Western society. We are work addicts obsessed with "doing" to the point where our human "beingness" (our spiritual side) suffers greatly. We are driven, but driving without ever refueling leaves us depleted. Sabbath offers the gift of replenishment.

PLAY AND PRAY

Many people view Sabbath as merely taking a break from their normal work activities. While that is certainly a part of it, it is not the full picture. Sabbath is *not* defined as not working; it means *playing*.

While we all pine for our once-per-year vacation, we are often much more comfortable with work than with play. How many of us have ever muttered the words, "I need a vacation from my vacation!" And that's because, even on vacation, it can be difficult for the average Westerner to truly relax. Our vacations have full, stressful itineraries and we load ourselves up with our favorite overindulgences. Unfortunately, this is far from magic for the soul.

Sabbath is a "play and pray" opportunity when you can take part in what delights you and strengthens your connection with the divine. And "pray" does *not* have to mean "go to church"—unless, of course, attending church or temple brings you great joy! If it does not, then don't even think about this as part of your Sabbath.

There are many ways to pray and many ways to play. Pick your favorites and devote time on your Sabbath day to them. That's the only real rule! The only parameter of Sabbath is *joy*. As Nelson states, "What intrigues, amazes, tickles your fancy, delights your senses, and casts you into an entirely new and unlimited world is the raw material of Sabbath."

Find Your Palace in Time

Time is the ultimate form of wealth in the modern world. It is common for Westerners to complain more about having no time than about having no money. Mostly, we are so busy trying to make money that we have little time to spend it. And because we work so hard during the week, our weekends become about who is the most efficient taskmaster and time manager. And Sunday, our supposed day of rest, has been hijacked by yardwork and laundry and grocery shopping and getting ready for the week and, likely, whatever work we brought home on Friday. Because time is the ultimate desire of the modern world, to dedicate an entire day to unplugging is considered a luxury, as it seemingly rebels against productivity. However, Sabbath is not a luxury, but a necessity.

Rabbi Abraham Joshua Heschel calls Sabbath a "palace in time." How nice does that sound? Remember that what we pay attention to grows, so if we consciously dedicate some of our time to generating a sense of awe and wonder to replenish our spirit, then our lives will inevitably be filled with more joy and more inspiration.

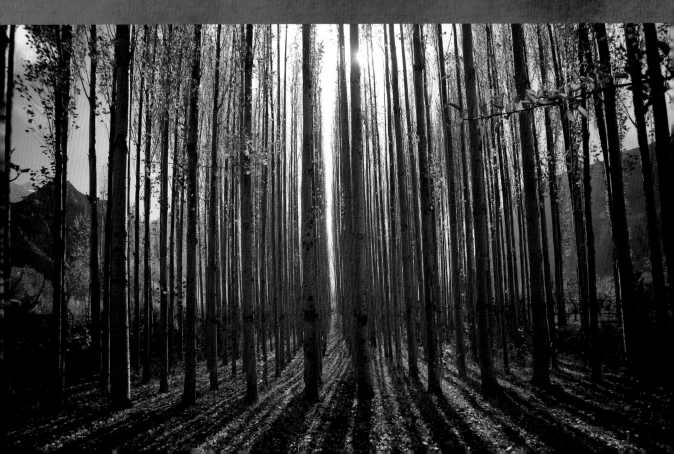

Sabbath Practices

The best way to begin formulating your Sabbath practice is to ask yourself: What brings me joy? What lights up my heart and soul? Below are some ideas to get (or give!) the most out of your Sabbath day.

FEAST

Eating good food is a great source of joy for many people, but the difference between "eating" and "feasting" is paramount for Sabbath. For example, imagine eating a five-star meal completely alone every night for the rest of your life. Sure, it would always taste delicious, but not being able to share the deliciousness with people you love would begin to wear on you and to feel empty.

To be fully enjoyed, a meal is best eaten in communion, which is where "feasting" comes in. The word *feast* means "a large meal, typically a celebratory one." And it's the word *celebratory* that makes feasting on Sabbath a great idea! Sharing food with those we love is a highly recommended activity on your day of joyful rest.

FAMILY FOCUS

Beyond sharing meals, Sabbath is meant to be communal in every aspect. In the modern day, some of us are close to our biological or chosen families and some of us are not. So, when we say "family focus," we mean spending focused time with those most dear to you. Connect in real and meaningful ways to those you love, whatever that looks like.

EXPLORE

The word *wonder* means a feeling of amazement and admiration, caused by something beautiful, remarkable, or unfamiliar. Socrates said that "wonder is the beginning of wisdom." Sabbath is a day to follow our curiosities and to explore the beautiful and unfamiliar. Whether reading up on a new subject or experiencing nature in some way, exploring your curiosities will ultimately lead to wonder and to expanded wisdom.

CREATE

At its core, spirituality *is* creativity. Spirit is creative and we are spirit. We are here on Earth to let spirit express itself through us. What will you create from the deepest well of love inside you? Will you sing? Paint? Write? Dance? Knit? Make a sandcastle with your kids? Whatever knocks on the door to your soul, let it out on Sabbath!

THANKS GIVING

God did not rest on the seventh day due to tiredness. God doesn't get tired! God rested to bask in the beauty of God's creation. And we are to do the same during our weekly Sabbath! We can offer gratitude for what we have created, and thus, what we have. Devote some time to counting your blessings each week and watch them multiply throughout the years.

VOLUNTEER

Service brings the ultimate form of joy. Giving back will connect you with gratitude and humility. Ask yourself, *In what ways can I serve my community that also lights me up?* It's important not to spend your Sabbath day volunteering out of a sense of obligation or piety, but because it brings you delight. So be sure to choose a way of giving back that really stirs your soul. Sabbath is an invitation to reconnect with your community and remember that, ultimately, we are here to learn to love one another unconditionally.

DIGITAL DETOX

This last point should go without saying, but in a tech-crazed world it is important to stress that Sabbath absolutely does not involve screen time of any kind. The whole point is to unplug from the mundane, and screens are one of the biggest perpetuators of all that madness. Sabbath is about tuning out of social media and tuning in to the soul magic inside of you.

"Those who have Sabbaths long for heaven, and those who long for heaven love Sabbaths."

—*Philip Henry*

Unplug a Little Every Day

You might not like this one, but it's very,
very vital to maintaining a healthy lifestyle:
keep your phone out of the bedroom at
night! Choose a time that the phone goes
off and is put away and stick to it. It's
not enough to just turn it off. Put it in
another room so that you are not tempted
to reach for it first thing in the morning.

Instead of scrolling through Instagram upon
waking, start your day right by flooding your
thoughts with gratitude, meditating, and
visualizing your perfect day in your mind.
Making the first few minutes of your morning
intentionally inspired will reap rewards for the
rest of the day. (And if you use your phone as
your alarm clock, don't use that as an excuse
to skip this important step! Go old school
and get yourself a bedside alarm clock.)

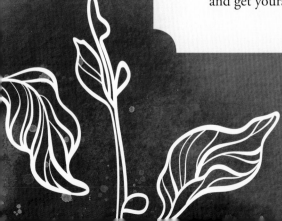

NUMEROLOGY

"Numerology is far more than a system of divination.
It is a language helping us understand spirit
and how it functions through humanity."

—*Divyaa Kummar*

We know: you hated math class. Bear with us for a moment. We
promise that a calculator is not needed to do numerology.

Numbers are the framework of the entire universe. All matter is, at its core, a
mathematical equation. Deeply linked to the subconscious mind, numbers are a sacred
language, the understanding of which is called numerology. Numerology is a method of
divination that uses numbers as symbols of different vibrational patterns. We can use this
system to discover deep truths about our personality and our purpose in this lifetime and
in lifetimes past.

PYTHAGORAS: MORE THAN JUST TRIANGLES

You probably remember the name Pythagoras and his theorem about triangles from high
school geometry class, but did you know this Greek philosopher is also considered the
father of numerology? Pythagoras, who famously said, "All is number," believed that
anything could be translated into a mathematical form and deciphered through the lens
of numerology. His method of assigning numerical values to letters became the basis for
the Pythagorean number system, which is used in modern numerology as well as tarot
and Qabalah. Pythagoras's followers also realized that adding up a series of odd numbers
beginning with the number 1 will always result in a square number. Numbers seem to
have an inherent power to balance out, create harmony, and function in a way that is
both predictable and mystical.

Calculating Your Numerology Chart

Just like you can create an astrological natal chart, you can also create a numerology chart using both your name on your birth certificate and your birth date. This is complex, because there are many different elements of a chart and reading how the numbers work together is truly an art, but you can calculate your life path number, expression, personality, and soul urge numbers using basic calculations. This is an easy and fun way to start working with numbers and seeing their significance in your life. (*Note:* If you've changed your name or don't use your given name at all, you can still calculate a numerology chart, just keep in mind that it could potentially be a bit off. Your birth name is coded with insight, and it is best to use that whenever possible for numerology purposes.)

Although there are various numerology chart systems, we prefer to use the Pythagorean system. This method assigns a number from 1 to 9 to each letter of the alphabet. All double-digit numbers are added together to get a single-digit number, from 1 to 9. The only double-digit numbers that are *not* added together are 11, 22, and 33, because they are "master numbers" and contain special significance. By adding the numerical values together, you can calculate a numerology chart using the steps below and then read the hidden messages in it (see pages 79-80 for the characteristics of each number).

1	2	3	4	5	6	7	8	9
A	B	C	D	E	F	G	H	I
J	K	L	M	N	O	P	Q	R
S	T	U	V	W	X	Y	Z	X

EXPRESSION NUMBER

Your expression number is also known as your destiny number and contains insight into your abilities, desires, and personal goals. It can also help you discover inherent traits. To calculate this number, use your full birth name and the Pythagorean numerology chart above. Add the individual digits of each letter of your name, and then keep adding the result to reduce the number down to a single digit or a master number.

Your expression number correlates with your life path number and is in relationship to your chart as a whole. You can learn more about what makes you tick through this number. Again, each number 1 to 9 contains a different meaning, as do the master numbers.

LIFE PATH NUMBER

Your life path number is the most important number in numerology. This number tells you, literally, what path your life will take (within the elasticity of free will, of course) and is reflective of who you are, who you will become, and what challenges you may face along your path. As with everything, there is a light and a shadow cast by your life path number, and you will be presented with opportunities to overcome the shadow and transmute it into light.

Life path numbers all contain different meanings and are from 1 to 9, plus the master numbers of 11, 22, and 33. To calculate your life path number, simply add up the numbers of your birth date individually, then reduce the number down to a single digit, save for in instances of a master number, which remains double digits. For example, May 10, 1986, would be:

$5 + 1 + 0 + 1 + 9 + 8 + 6 = 30$; $3 + 0 = 3$. This is a 3 life path number.

PERSONALITY NUMBER

Your personality number is calculated using only the consonants in your name and adding them up with the same process as your expression number. This is your outward-facing persona and the first impression people see. People will most likely associate you more with your personality number than your life path number, because it's what you allow people to see, while the core of yourself will only ever be truly known by you.

Discovering this number can be enlightening in the sense that you'll understand more about your interactions with people, their reactions to you, and your reactions in certain situations. If you've been wondering why someone thinks you're a certain way, the answer is likely hiding in your personality number.

SOUL URGE NUMBER

Also referred to as the "heart's desire" number, your soul urge number symbolizes a reflection of your inner world, your emotions, and your fears. Calculating this number can reveal things about you that you were never aware of, but that can be quite affirming. Much of our soul urge number is known innately because it is often what we repress within ourselves or rationalize away from (this is called the golden shadow, which you can learn more about in the shadow work chapter). The heart is not logical, and discovering this number can lead to a deeper understanding of the self.

To calculate this number, use only the vowels in your name, and the same system as the personality and expression numbers. The interesting correlation between this number, its significance, and vowels is that in many ancient cultures, vowels are chanted and used in sound healing to reach higher states of consciousness. This is completely in line with this number's association with the heart's desire.

BIRTH DAY NUMBER

The day you are born holds incredible significance, of course. This number holds the key to your destiny and is calculated using the number of the day you were born. If you were born on the 24th, for example, you add 2 + 4 = 6. When looked at in relation to your entire numerology chart, the birth day number is akin to a compass.

"The very numbers you use in counting are more than you take them for. They are at the same time mythological entities (for the Pythagoreans they were even divine), but you are certainly unaware of this when you use numbers for a practical purpose."

—*Carl Jung*, THE SYMBOLIC LIFE

The Meaning of the Numbers

1 You're a natural leader and blessed with motivation, enthusiasm, and drive. Put yourself out there and you'll be the most fulfilled. The shadow side of 1 can cause alienation from loved ones and society in pursuit of success.

2 You're a lover by nature and easily connect with others on a deep level. You bring harmony and love to situations, but you can easily take on the problems of others with your empathetic nature.

3 You're the boss and a powerhouse who needs to be seen and known. Characterized by beauty, eccentricity, and fame, you love to share your inner calling with the world on a grand scale. It's vital to retain your sense of wonder so as not to fall into depression or give up on your calling.

4 Strong, dependable, and balanced, you're the pillar of your community. You are practical, trustworthy, hardworking, and resourceful. Although your intentions are always pure, you can be easily taken advantage of or be misunderstood as a martyr or tyrant.

5 Curious, intelligent, and highly philosophical, you are very cerebral. You learn by being hands-on and many come to you for your wisdom. You can, however, become very self-absorbed and push people away, preventing long-lasting bonds from forming.

6 A natural caregiver, you feel most satisfied when you are serving in a dedicated way to a person or a cause. It is easy for you to lose yourself in serving others and feel as if you are enslaved.

7 You are an analytical and deep thinker who loves to discover how it all works and what it all means. This can, however, fall into overthinking and questioning everything. It's important for you to learn to trust your own head and heart.

8 The number of power and prosperity means you are driven to achieve but on a deep and meaningful level. By learning to bounce back from life's challenges, you'll be able to embody your infinite power.

Magic vs. Magick

The *k* in *magick* is used in relation to the occult and differentiates it from the sideshow magic of illusion. The occult, which uses mystical, supernatural, or magickal powers, is the knowledge of the hidden. The occult is not dark or black magick, nor is it satanic.

9 You are an old soul and the embodiment of wisdom. Healing the world is your mission and you have the insight to do it. On the shadow side, however, you can come across as condescending or as a "know it all."

10 * You are radiance personified. Because 10 is a number of brilliance, potential, and ease, you are able to call in all you desire with a rare and precise accuracy. However, 10 is a number of extremes and you can easily get caught in the power of 1, or the abyss of 0.

*The Qabalist (an esoteric method, discipline, and school of thought in Jewish mysticism) numerology tradition is the only one where 10 is not reduced to 1, making modern interpretations of this life path number specific to that philosophy alone.

11 This master number means you are on a search for enlightenment. You easily swing from challenge to growth and are often the "wounded healer" who has experienced hardship and turns it around to help others. Because of this journey, you may have a chip on your shoulder that can hold you back from shining your light.

22 You are a master manifester and designer of life. You are both visionary and practical and have unique ideas. It may take you your entire life to embody your divinity, and you can easily get lost in your comfort zone.

33 The most prominent of master numbers, and also the rarest, 33 means you are the "teacher" and the closest to the divine, or "Christ Consciousness." You are a selfless caregiver, highly nurturing and compassionate. The shadow side means you can be high strung, controlling, or overemotional.

Numbers and Synchronicity

The first rule of numerology is that there are no coincidences. Beyond your personal chart and the numbers associated with your name and birthday, there are numbers all around us that contain significance, messages, and guidance.

If you're well versed in modern mysticism, then you've likely heard about the magick of repeating numbers and sequences of numbers, such as 1111, 222, 444, 1234, and so on. Modern mystics go wild for synchronicities in numbers because it makes us feel like we aren't alone and like there is a lot of activity happening "beyond the veil" to support us on our journey.

Often referred to as "angel numbers," numbers that you see over and over throughout the day—or that show on the clock when you wake up in the middle of the night—bear a message from the world of spirit. The spiritual realm loves to communicate through technology, and clocks are one of the easiest ways to catch our attention with numbers.

There are many explanations of what sequences of numbers mean, but we think it's best to listen to your intuition and to try to decipher the message on your own. For example, the number 15 may have great significance to you, and seeing it will mean something different to you than to someone else.

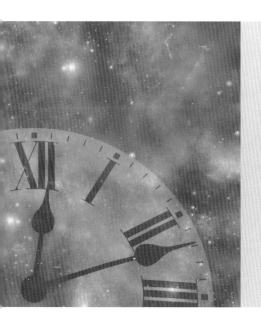

Look for the Signs

Start paying attention to the numbers that you see frequently. Keep a journal for noting when a number keeps popping up, and record where it's happening and what you're thinking about at the time. Avoid going straight to Google for the number's meaning; instead, tap into your intuition. This is a wonderful way to connect with the mystical properties of numbers and to begin to decipher messages that are meant specifically for you. You'll be surprised by how much we are guided by these signs when we are open to them. The universe loves to co-create with us.

CEREMONIAL MAGICK

"There is no greater power than the one others do not believe you possess."

—*Luis Marques,* Book of Orion

This is not a chapter about bubbling cauldrons, broomsticks, and pointy hats, or a recap of Harry Potter's most famous spells. This is about the magick that resides within each of us, and which you can learn to harness with intention. It does involve making a cool wand, though, so read on!

For as long as there have been humans, there has been some form of magick. We have always been curious about the natural world, and magick is the way in which we wield our wands to bring intention to manifestation. Facilitated by alchemists, witches, wizards, high priestesses, sorcerers, mystics, sages, and the like, magick has been used for both good and evil for millennia. Magick was first used to facilitate good—for protection and to connect with the unseen world of spirit. However, as the power of magick grew, so did the potential for it to go into darkness. As with everything, duality is present in magick, too.

"Words and magic were in the beginning one and the same thing, and even today words retain much of their magical power."

—*Sigmund Freud,* Introductory Lectures on Psychoanalysis

What Is "Ceremonial Magick"?

Magick is often confused with witchcraft, vodoo, paganism, shamanism, and mysticism. While those mystical practices all do *use* magick, what we are referring to is something different. Ceremonial magick is commonly divided into two realms: "low magick," which is more folk magick or nature magick and works with herbs, the seasons, the elements, and astrology, and "high magick," which is more of an art and science that works with energetic principles of the universe. In ancient times, this form of magick was typically reserved for philosophers, scholars, and intellectuals and was hidden behind "mystery schools." In both realms, however, ceremonial magick uses specific rituals and invocations to call upon the spirit world and to shift energy.

Magick is not an illusion on a Las Vegas stage, nor is it dark and evil (although some people use it for dark or evil purposes). It is a creative force that uses the laws of the natural and supernatural worlds to alter reality and to manifest desires. Through ceremonial magick, we remember our connection to nature, to ceremony and ritual, and to the power of the focused and intentional mind to co-create with spirit. Ceremonial magick involves tarot, numerology, Western astrology, ritual, alchemy, tantra, hermeticism, and the Qabalah.

A Brief History of Magick

In their own unique ways, every ancient culture possessed and utilized a form of magick—which was originally used to heal, not to curse. Magick follows the natural laws of the universe, including, most importantly, the power of the mind. In ancient times, magick and religion coexisted with very little tension; the two worked together in tandem. Magick was merely a part of everyday life and was used in religious rituals.

The word *magic,* or *magick,* comes from the Asyro-Babylonian civilizations, where the highest priests were called magi and practiced a "religion" later called magick. Magi were known to use astronomy/astrology, alchemy, and other forms of esoteric knowledge in their magickal practices. We know that magi were respected as "wise men," as is evidenced by the three wise men who brought gifts to baby Jesus, who were famously called "the magi."

How to Do Ceremonial Magick

You don't have to be part of a coven to do ceremonial magick, although surrounding yourself with like-minded people who understand this sacred art is definitely helpful. Magick is both active and passive, and for any sort of work or magick to be made manifest, an active factor (masculine energy) and a passive factor (feminine energy) must work together. A ceremony or ritual is active, and the surrender and release of the outcome is passive. If you set an intention, cast a spell, or invoke a deity, the real magick is in the release of attachment to a specific result and being open to allowing magick to provide the best possible outcome. Surrendering to the power of the subconscious mind to co-create with spirit is the real magick wand!

PURIFICATION

The first step is to prepare yourself for spiritual work through ritual purification. In the past, practitioners would purify themselves through a rigorous diet, meditation, cleansing the body, fasting, prayer, and sexual abstinence. Or you can take a ceremonial bath to purify your mind and body. You may wish to include crystals (see page 24), essential oils (see page 12), or incense (see page 18) in your ritual bath.

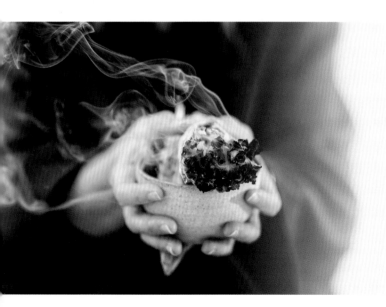

You can also put on a ceremonial robe before beginning your ritual. Doing so symbolizes your clear frame of mind and pure intention.

THE MAGICK CIRCLE

Now it's time to cast a magick circle. This defines your space and allows you to set your intention for magick to happen. If you are outside, draw a circle on the ground with chalk, paint, or rock salt. If you are inside, such as in your living room, you can use a long rope or cord. Make sure the circle remains intact and is not broken in any point along its line. This is also a great time to use crystals to enhance the vibrational energy of the space (see page 24). Stand inside the circle with any participants who are with you. The circle now contains and focuses your collective energy, protects the participants, and keeps out unwanted vibes.

Purify the magick circle with the four elements: fire, air, water, and earth. The dagger that is used in the banishing ritual (see below) is associated with the element of fire, so purification is traditionally done with the remaining three elements, using incense to symbolize air, water for water, and salt to symbolize earth. Light incense and use a feather to waft the smoke around the magick circle. Next, sprinkle water and then salt around the circle.

BANISHING

Now it's time to banish any malevolent forces that may interfere with your ritual. This forms a protective barrier and facilitates a positive outcome. A common method, known as the Lesser Banishing Ritual of the Pentagram, uses a pentagram, a five-pointed star with the point facing up.

1. Using a magickal implement or "weapon," such as a ceremonial dagger or sword, "draw" the pentagram in the air at each of the four cardinal points, starting in the east and moving clockwise to south, then west, then north. This is also a process of invoking the elemental guardians of the four directions, known as "calling the quarters."

2. At each cardinal point, holding your magickal implement straight in front of you, draw the pentagram starting from the lower left, following the diagram below. As you do this, visualize each line and then the final star as glowing white lines.

3. At the same time, you can chant an incantation or an intention. Some people chant sacred names of God, the names of the archangels, or a mantra.

4. Keep your arm up so that each new pentagram you draw is connected to the next and creates a strong barrier all around your circle.

5. Visualize these vibrantly glowing pentagrams and their connecting lines and feel the pulsing energy keeping you safe. If you wish, you can visualize the circle of pentagrams moving out beyond the space of your circle to encompass a greater area of protection, such as your home.

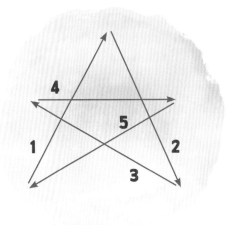

CONSECRATION

In this part of the ceremony, announce that you dedicate the ritual instrument (such as a wand) or your space (such as the magick circle) to the purpose at hand: summoning spirit for the highest good.

INVOCATION

Now it is time to call up, or invoke, spirit. This could be a god or goddess, an entity, or a particular type of energy that you wish to manifest. Remember that you are summoning spirit for the highest good of all concerned.

DIVINE SACRAMENTS

Many magick rituals involve imbuing ordinary objects, usually food and drink, with sacred energy and then consuming them. Thus, you become infused with the divine properties embodied in the sacred object. The most common objects used for this part of the ritual are flat cakes (often referred to as "Cake of Light") and wine.

DIVINATION

You may wish to use divination tools, such as tarot cards (see page 180), numerology (see page 74), or astrology (see page 112), in your ritual in order to obtain guidance from the universal intelligence. This knowledge, or divine intuition, is meant to help you gain insight on the path to the higher self.

MAGICKAL RECORD

A magickal record is essentially a journal where you keep track of the details of your rituals, experiences, and ideas. This can help you determine the effectiveness of various procedures and their eventual outcomes.

While I was at a yoga retreat, the teacher took us to a nearby lake, and we stood on the shore and made a magick circle. Then the teacher invoked the four directions. While we were busy chanting and drumming, he faced the lake and stretched his arms out wide. A stiff breeze began blowing up off the lake. Within minutes it was so strong that it drowned out our chanting, kicking up sand and bending branches on the trees. A few minutes later, the wind calmed to a gentle breeze and then completely stopped. We were transfixed.

—*Nick, 27*

MAGICKAL IMPLEMENTS

Every magician needs a wand, right? To perform your magickal rituals, you'll need not only a wand but also a collection of magickal implements. These are often referred to as magickal "weapons," but they are really instruments that are used to bring about intentional change, such as a wand or sword. These are your sacred items, so consecrate them for use in ceremonial magick. You might hold your magickal implements and invoke spirit to help you use them for the highest good, and you can purify them with fire, air (using incense), water, and earth (using salt).

The four elemental tools are the dagger (or spear), wand, pentacle, and cup or chalice. These tools correspond to the four weapons of significance in Celtic myth—the sword, the spear, the shield, and the cauldron (and/or grail). They also appear in tarot decks as the four card suits: swords, wands, pentacles, and cups. You can buy these items from a magick shop (there are many online!) or make your own.

DAGGER

In ceremonial magick, this tool is known as an athame. It is a black-handled ceremonial knife generally used in banishing rituals to expel unwanted energy from your magick circle (see page 85). You'll use the dagger to channel and direct energy for the highest good during your rituals. One thing you need to know about athames: Never touch another person's athame without permission. It is considered an offensive invasion of personal space and requires the person to rededicate and reconsecrate the athame.

WAND

A wand used for magick is generally made of wood, with oak and hazel being two of the most common. Wands are traditionally used to invite spirit and angels and for other forms of spellcasting. They are associated with the element of air. In tarot cards, the suit of wands is usually signified as a tree branch or stick, reflecting its association with nature.

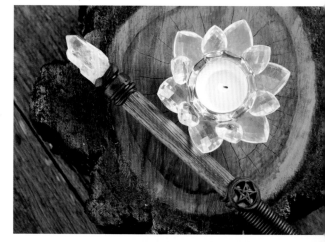

How to Make Your Own Wand

1. Find a branch that is the size and shape you want. About the width of your thumb and the length of your forearm are good size guidelines, but choose a branch that feels good in your hand. **Branches collected after a violent storm also make powerful wands.**

2. Set your branch in a dry place with good circulation to cure for about a month.

3. Select a crystal that corresponds to your wand's specific use (see page 24). Place the crystal at the tip of your wand to amplify its energy, using copper or silver wire, both good conductors of energy, to attach the crystal.

4. Again using copper or silver wire, attach a stone or other object at the base of the wand to ground and store energy.

5. If you wish to decorate your wand, elements from nature, such as acorns and pinecones, are good choices. You can also use beads in colors that correspond to your specific purpose (see page 34).

6. Cleanse all the items you'll be using in your wand so that their energy will be pure. See page 31 for how to cleanse items for ritual use.

7. You can strip the bark or leave it on. You can sand the wand smooth or leave it rough.

8. Use a wood-burning tool, carving tools, or paint to decorate your wand with any symbols you wish.

9. If you wish, varnish or stain your wand, and wrap the handle with ribbons or leather, to make it more comfortable to hold. You can also drill a hole in the handle and run a ribbon through it as a wrist strap.

10. Once your wand is complete, charge it into your service. You can give it a general charge (e.g., "I charge this wand to help me work with spirit for the highest good of all concerned") or a specific charge (e.g., to heal or attract loving energy). If you wish, give your wand a name that embodies your intention for it.

11. Practice sending energy through your wand into objects. Wave your wand and visualize stars streaming from the tip.

PENTACLE

In magick, a pentacle is a talisman that can incorporate many different symbols or characters. It is often drawn on a circular piece of parchment, paper, or cloth, or on a metal disk. Traditionally, these are hung around the neck to provide protection to the wearer. The pentacle is associated with the element of earth.

CUP OR CHALICE

This is a goblet used to hold wine during rituals. The chalice, a feminine principle, is associated with water and the moon. It is often used in combination with the athame, which is considered a masculine principle and is associated with the element of fire and the sun. The union of these two implements represents the union of opposites in sacred marriage: male and female, sun and moon, fire and water. This rite is done by dipping the athame into the chalice to bless the wine, a ritual also known as the Great Rite.

Other Magickal Objects

- For the purposes of ceremonial magick, practitioners usually include *Abramelin oil*, a ceremonial oil blended with aromatic plants. The historical blend included various proportions of myrrh, cinnamon, calamus, and cassia steeped in olive oil. Today, people use essential oils instead of plant material to make Abramelin oil. (See the chapter on aromatherapy for more information on using essential oils.)

- Small *oil lamps* made of stone, metal, or ceramic are used to hold the ceremonial oil.

- *Bells* are used to banish unwanted energy and to attune the energy within the magick circle. The clear, healing tone of the bell affects energy on a physical, emotional, and spiritual level (see the chapter on sound healing for more information).

- A *censer* is used to burn incense during a ceremonial ritual. (See the chapter on aromatherapy for more information on using incense.)

- A *grimoire* is a book of spells and magick incantations. Many grimoires are themselves believed to be imbued with magick. Select a book that calls to you and use it to create ceremonial magick that is in the highest good.

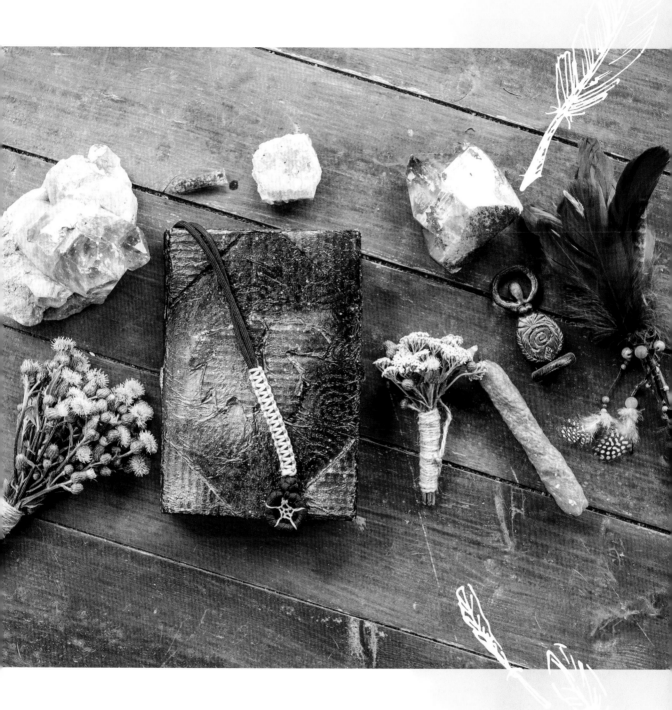

SACRED TRAVEL

"Don't tell me how educated you are,
tell me how much you traveled."

—*Mohammad*

An age-old tradition, sacred travel—or pilgrimage—is an important
part of every spiritual path. This devotional practice consists of a long
journey, usually on foot, toward a significant and meaningful destination.
It is a transformational experience, where you leave your limited frame
of reference—your home, your identity, the roles you play in your
family—and journey toward an expansive unknown and your higher self.
The fact that such a journey most often takes place in the presence of
hundreds of thousands of others heightens its spiritual significance.

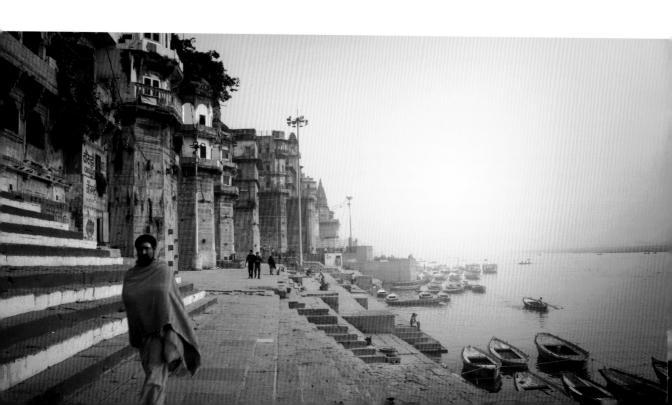

The Purpose of a Pilgrimage

A pilgrimage offers spiritual seekers two things: an inward journey
and outward discipline. Pilgrimage requires discipline and
devotion to uncovering our highest, most authentic selves.

The physical destination for the modern mystic doesn't really matter; it's the "back
to oneself" intention that is the core of any pilgrimage. Back to your own innate
divinity. Back to your life's purpose. Back to your highest, soulful, magickal self. For
transformation, we often have to go away in order to come home to our true selves.

> "The purpose of a pilgrimage is about setting
> aside a long period of time in which the only
> focus is to be the matters of the soul. Many
> believe a pilgrimage is about going away,
> but it isn't; it is about coming home."
>
> —*L. M. Browning*, Seasons of Contemplation

Your personal pilgrimage does *not* have to be extreme or far-reaching. It only must
be meaningful to *you*. No one else needs to understand it; it just has to feel right in your
heart, meant for no one but *you*.

While traditionally pilgrimages were undertaken on foot or on horseback, and many
still are, the modern pilgrim can also choose to bike, drive, ride a train, sail, or fly. Want
to repurpose an old VW bus and journey across every state in the USA? Pilgrimage.
Want to sail around the world for a year? Pilgrimage. Want to cycle through Europe to
various monasteries? Pilgrimage. Whatever you want to commit to that moves you from
point A to point B and stirs your soul is a pilgrimage. A profound-to-you destination or
goal is required, but, as always, the true point is the journey.

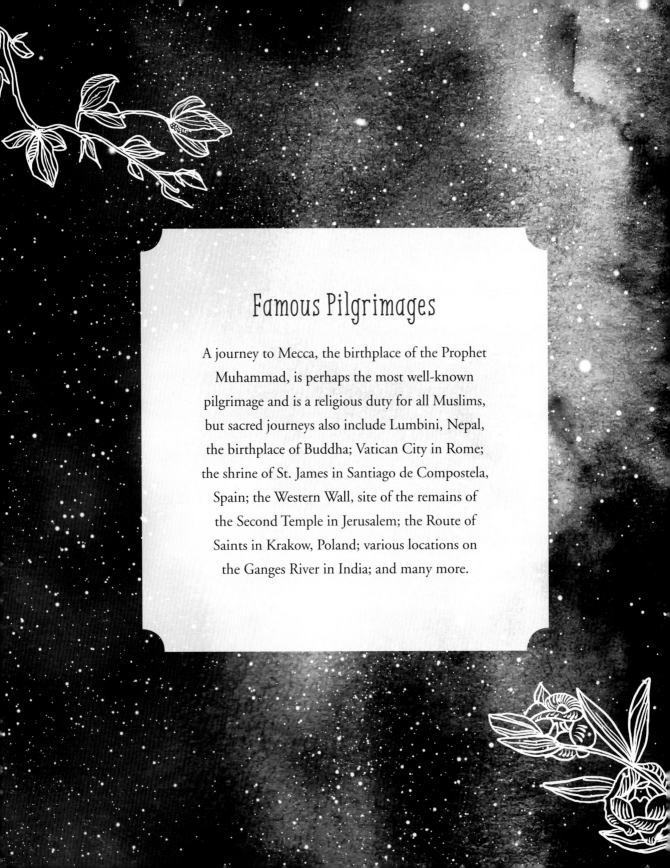

Famous Pilgrimages

A journey to Mecca, the birthplace of the Prophet
Muhammad, is perhaps the most well-known
pilgrimage and is a religious duty for all Muslims,
but sacred journeys also include Lumbini, Nepal,
the birthplace of Buddha; Vatican City in Rome;
the shrine of St. James in Santiago de Compostela,
Spain; the Western Wall, site of the remains of
the Second Temple in Jerusalem; the Route of
Saints in Krakow, Poland; various locations on
the Ganges River in India; and many more.

Three Historical Pilgrimages That Resonate Today

While customizing your pilgrimage to your own soul's desire is vital,
numerous traditional pilgrimage routes are still relevant to many. Hundreds
of thousands of modern seekers choose to stick to the ancient pilgrimages
that will always hold so much power. Here are our top picks.

CAMINO DE SANTIAGO

Also known as the Way of Saint James, this is one of the most popular pilgrimages in
Europe today. The history goes that the body of Saint James the Apostle was discovered
by a shepherd in a field in Galicia, Spain, back in the ninth century. King Alfonso II
then had a small chapel built in this holy place (later commissioning a larger temple),
and it has since attracted pilgrims from all over the world. Prior to the discovery of Saint
James's body, the Camino de Santiago was known as a route that the ancients walked to
follow the path of the Milky Way. The destination, Finisterre, was believed to be the end
of the world, as well as a magical place where the living could get closest to "the other
side"—the land of the dead. Travelers of this road today often tell stories of personal
transformation and spiritual awakening.

Many years ago, I went to visit Tikal, a huge archeological site of the pre-Columbian
Maya civilization. One evening, with a few friends and a guide, we hiked with flashlights
through the jungle to get to the main complex of temples. We climbed to the top of
the largest temple, up the steep stairs, and sat at the top, on the moss-covered rock,
gazing at the site spread before us and the brilliant stars above. The howler monkeys
began their nocturnal calls. The ground felt holy, alive with hundreds of souls who
had lived and died there and participated in their sacred rituals of games and human
sacrifice. It was a deeply spiritual experience that still informs my journey to this day.

—Micha, 67

BODHGAYA

Bodhgaya in Bihar—whose famous fig tree is said to have been where the Buddha meditated for seven days and ultimately attained enlightenment—is the holiest site of Buddhism today. The journey there is considered the most sacred pilgrimage to Buddhists as well as people of various faiths interested in Buddhist philosophy. The site is also used for performing rites for departed ancestors, keeping the spirit of the place alive and palpable.

JERUSALEM

The capital city of Israel has attracted droves of pilgrims ever since the original pilgrims, the three wise men, made the journey. Considered the world's holiest city, Jerusalem has historical and spiritual roots for Muslims, Jews, and Christians. For the biblically inclined, this pilgrimage takes you to Bethlehem, Capernaum, Nazareth, Mount Zion, and Cana, allowing you to walk the very paths that Jesus walked.

Other Pilgrimage Ideas

Here are some other sources of inspiration for pilgrimage sites:

- **PLACES STEEPED IN MYSTERY:** Stonehenge in England, the Richart Structure in Mauritania, Lines of Nazca in Peru, and the Oracle of Delphi in Greece.

- **ANCIENT RUINS:** Machu Picchu in Peru, the Great Pyramids in Egypt, Tulum in Mexico, or Angkor Wat in Cambodia.

- **ANCIENT TEMPLES AND CHURCHES:** Rosslyn Chapel in Scotland, Boudhanath Stupa in Nepal, rock-hewn churches in Ethiopia, and Taktsang monastery in Bhutan.

- **PLACES WHERE THERE IS BELIEVED TO BE SPECIAL ENERGY OR WHERE ANCIENT RITES TOOK PLACE:** Stone circles, crop circles, healing waters, and sacred mountains.

- **LOCALES OF GREAT NATURAL BEAUTY:** Ayers Rock in Australia, Devils Tower in Wyoming, or Victoria Falls in Zambia and Zimbabwe.

- **PLACES THAT ARE REMOTE AND OFF THE GRID:** The Arctic, Siberia, or Easter Island.

- **THE WILDERNESS:** Hiking, kayaking, or canoeing to places not frequented by others.

- **A DARK SKY PRESERVE:** A place where you can view the Milky Way and constellations you've never seen before. To find a dark sky preserve, go to www.darksky.org/our-work/conservation/idsp/parks.

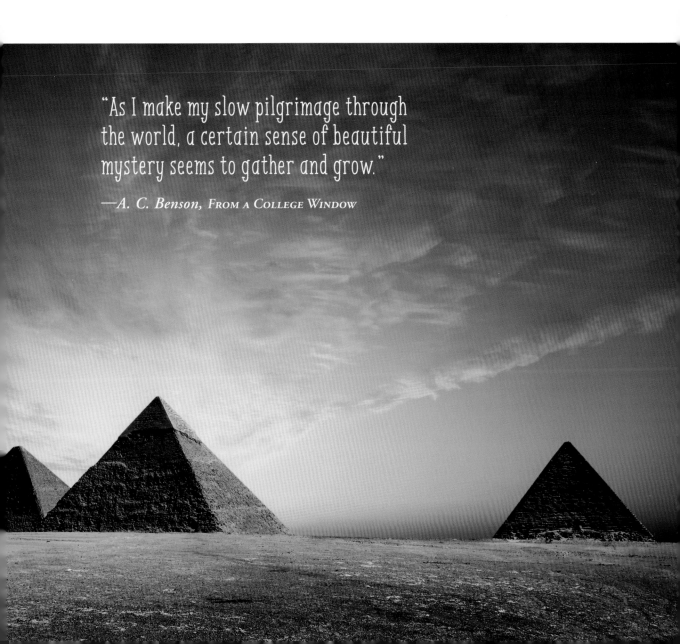

"As I make my slow pilgrimage through the world, a certain sense of beautiful mystery seems to gather and grow."

—A. C. Benson, FROM A COLLEGE WINDOW

I became an avid skygazer at a young age. One year I went to Namibia, one of the darkest countries in the world. Out in the desert I gazed up at the brightest sky I had ever seen. Distinctly visible were a huge swath of the Milky Way, the Southern Cross, nebulae, and constellations I had never seen before. It was overwhelming. I have never felt so small yet so connected to the universe. I felt my ego dissolving and merging with the Great Consciousness.

—*Ali, 45*

Intuitive Travel

Sacred travel is the way to gather and grow yourself in a world that often does the opposite to us, leaving us feeling scattered and withered. It's a way to understand what truly has value in our life, and what does not. And it's a way to put our intuition ahead of our logic, allowing us to see things from another perspective.

The difference between a standard vacation and sacred travel can be summed up exactly by the word *intuition*. Intuitive travel does not involve rigid itineraries and maps; it does not involve knowing everything before you step out the door and onto the plane, train, or automobile. In fact, the very purpose of intuitive travel is to *not* know what you are looking for at all. It's about letting go of your addiction to control, surrendering to the higher guidance of your soul, and being open to the best possibilities for you. The beautiful mystery is what you're after, and the only compass you need for that is the compass of your soul. Practicing intuitive travel means you let your spirit guide you. And when you do that, you'll often be awestruck by the places you end up.

> "A good traveler has no fixed plans
> and is not intent on arriving."
>
> —*Lao Tzu, Tao Te Ching*

So, leave aside the Google maps and let the whispers of your soul be your guiding light. Let your internal compass guide you, even if just for a day. Ask your soul where it wants to go, which turn to take, and invite the right people across your path. Go with what *feels good* in your heart, always.

Intuitive travel also offers the huge benefit of meeting other spiritually inclined people. Like going to the gym with a buddy rather than alone, our spiritual "workouts" greatly improve when we have friends and community to encourage us along the way. Having a support system in your spiritual practice is vital. Intuitive travel that is based in trust in spirit brings you the people you need to meet, exactly when you need them—typically inspiring you to open your heart and mind more and more to your true self. We've never heard of one person who has gone on a spiritual pilgrimage and did not meet forever "soul mate" friends.

Re-treat Yo'self!

In a modern world brimming with stress, retreats of all kinds are rising in popularity. Whether you are interested in yoga, nutrition, developing your intuitive abilities, or something else, there is a retreat for you out there! Retreats are considered modern-day pilgrimages, as you are journeying to a sacred space, away from your everyday, mundane activities, with the intention of elevating your soul. And you're meeting like-minded friends for life. If your soul is calling out for a retreat to dive deeper into your spiritual journey, a solid place to find your perfect spiritual retreat is www.spiritual.directory.

YOGA

> *"Yoga is the journey of the self,*
> *through the self, to the self."*
>
> —*Bhagavad Gita*

Get ready for a mind blow if yoga sparks thoughts of expensive yoga mats and pants, retreats in Costa Rica, or catching that one-hour intro class at your gym. The original yogic philosophy, reverence, and wisdom has been lost in translation in our modern capitalistic world. When we reconnect with the roots of yoga and what it stands for, this practice can really perform the wonders it's meant to impart to the health of our bodies, minds, and souls.

We practice yoga to get out of our head, to get into our body, and to better manage the daily stress and tight muscles that our go-go-go society produces. While this is all well and good, yoga is meant to be a holistic lifestyle rather than a simple hour-a-week workout at your local gym or yoga studio in the tightest, most expensive yoga pants.

The widespread adoption and near obsession with yoga in the West has truly done a lot of good for millions of people. However, when we get too far from the roots of a profound practice like yoga, it's easy to forget the *why* and get lost in the matching yoga outfits and seemingly endless festivals and retreats. Yoga is bigger—and more profound—than that. Yoga is self-healing, strengthening, connecting, humbling, expansive. Yoga is the invocation of pure spirit.

Yoga is self-mastery and self-realization, and it extends far beyond the movements on the mat. **The yogic path is living our lives as if we are always on the mat**, in every aspect of life. This cultivates a life of self-awareness, nonattachment, devotion, perspective, and reverence. And while the physical aspect of yoga will inevitably cultivate fitness, the original yogic sciences place a larger emphasis on the fitness of the mind. When the mind is fit, life will flow, and the body will be a vibrant and healthy vessel in which to experience the world within and around it—and that's precisely the goal of our human existence.

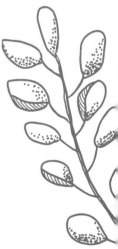

Ancient vs. Modern Yoga

Yoga originated in a large body of ancient texts from India, called the *Vedas*, nearly 5,000 years ago and laid a foundation on which all Indian culture was built. The philosophy of yoga was further described in the *Bhagavad Gita*, an ancient Indian text that became an important work of Hindu tradition.

The word *yoga* comes from the Sanskrit word *yuj*, which can be translated into "yoking" or "union" and refers to union of the individual self and the universal self. Yoga is first a spiritual practice; it was originally used to prime the body for long periods of sitting in meditation. But to fully embody the intention and potential of yoga for self-actualization, we must first understand that the *asanas*, or poses, are only one part of yoga.

Asanas weren't even part of yoga until the Indian sage Patanjali wrote *The Yoga Sutras* around 200 BCE. This text is the basis for the contemporary version of yoga we know today. Asanas were added to the practice of yoga to help the body integrate the spiritual journey of yoga. *Sutra* means "thread" or "weave," and it points to the connection between body, mind, and spirit through meaningful movement.

Ancient yoga was a spiritual system with the goal of achieving self-mastery and self-realization in order to ultimately unite with the divine. Modern yoga, by contrast, is heavily focused on the physical poses and views the spiritual as a secondary benefit of healing the physical body. When we lose the core of the spiritual practice, it is difficult to experience the incredibly comprehensive benefits of yoga that our ancestors did.

The modern mystic must *dig deeper*. We can establish a whole and intentional practice by understanding the roots of yoga and developing ways to incorporate the true path and spirituality of yoga in our daily life. This doesn't mean that you have to leave your favorite yoga studio, only that you should be more conscious of what yoga actually *is*, and more importantly, what it *isn't*.

"Yoga is the progressive settling of the mind into silence. When the mind is settled, we are established in our own essential state, which is unbounded consciousness. Our essential nature is usually overshadowed by the activity of the mind."

—*Patanjali*, THE YOGA SUTRAS

A Transformative Personal Journey: The Eight Limbs of Yoga

We can reconnect to the original spirit of yoga and bring this understanding into our modern practice by starting with what is called "the eight limbs of yoga." In order to merge into oneness, where there is no fear or suffering and love is the constant state of being, we must move through the eight limbs of yoga. This practice is referred to as raja yoga, or "the royal path."

The eight limbs of yoga come from *The Yoga Sutras* and encompass our entire world, within us and outside of us. The number eight in numerology signifies balance and prosperity and is the great karmic equalizer. It's not a coincidence (because there aren't any!) that this is also the number of "steps" to reach supreme and absolute oneness with all.

The goal of yoga is to still the mind so that we can merge into the oneness of our soul and the infinite universe. The mind is a powerful thing, and when left to its own devices, can be incredibly destructive—thank you, ego, for that! The yogic lifestyle, as opposed to the once-per-week workout, stills the mind so that the spirit and soul can fly free without egoic inhibition.

This yogic path of self-development is a personal journey that addresses the multifaceted parts of life and challenges you to look at your light and your darkness with compassion and a lack of judgment.

1. YAMAS (SELF-CONTROL)

The journey to oneness begins with yamas, which means "self-control" and is the moral and ethical compass upon which life and personal development are based. How we relate to the world will affect all of life and how we treat others. Within the yamas, there are five principles:

    a. Ahimsa: Nonviolence to self or others

    b. Satya: Truthfulness with self, others, and the universe

    c. Asteya: Non-stealing in form of materials or time/energy

    d. Brahmacharya: Non-indulgence of human, sensory pleasures

    e. Aparigraha: Non-possessiveness or attachment to material and worldly things

2. NIYAMAS (MORAL OBSERVANCE)

This step is where we turn our attention inward and focus on how we relate to ourselves. Self-discipline, self-development, and personal standards are described in the *niyamas*, which means "moral observance." Within the niyamas, there are five principles:

    a. Saucha: Cleanliness and purity of mind, body, and spirit

    b. Santosha: Contentment and being satisfied and grateful for what we have

    c. Tapas: Austerity and self-discipline over senses and desires

    d. Svadhyaya: Self-study and awareness of our patterns, beliefs, and purpose

    e. Ishvara Pranidhana: Surrender to, and connection with, personal divinity

3. ASANA (POSTURES)

This is the movement part of the yogic path and helps move energy, strengthens the body for the purpose of clear meditation, clears physical and energetic blockages, and connects us deeply within to the source of all life. *Asana* means "to sit," and helps keep the body's vital energy flowing.

The order of the path is progressive, so the first two limbs have to be mastered and integrated before moving on. Asana is an important way to integrate the first two and prepare for the remaining five limbs.

4. PRANAYAMA (BREATHWORK)

Breath is the source of life and energy. *Prana* means "vital life force" and yama means "vehicle" or "control." It is through conscious control of our life force— our breath—that we can connect deeply and ascend to our highest potential. When we expand our energy through breathing techniques, our prana will flow vibrantly through our body with ease, literally breathing life into areas that are blocked or stuck and offering the deepest healing.

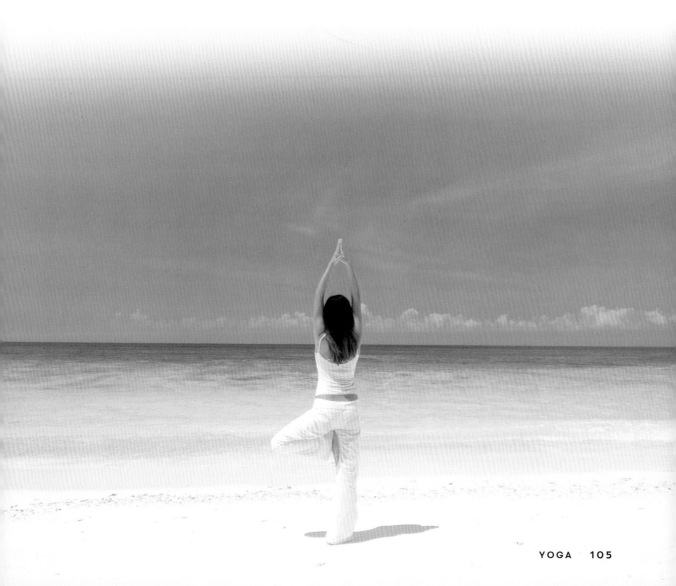

5. PRATAYAHRA (WITHDRAWAL FROM THE SENSES)

The mind is stimulated by external senses—touch, taste, smell, sound, and feeling. Our senses conjure a reaction and association/attachment that can be distracting. Pratyahara teaches withdrawal from the senses so attention can go inward. This can be done by closing the eyes in meditation, using ear plugs during asana, or even using a blindfold in asana. We can train the brain to operate without stimulation, or in the case of unavoidable stimulation, be unaffected by it.

6. DHARANA (FOCUS IN THE MIND)

Once we've withdrawn from the senses, we can progress to a singular point of focus. Dharana is concentration and the reward of the first five limbs. This control of the mind is the precursor for meditation but must be mastered before we can meditate with purpose. To help quiet the mind after sensory deprivation, we can use a word or a mantra to bring the attention of the mind to one point. By having something to concentrate on, the mind will begin to still, and after sustained periods of dharana, we can then naturally move into meditation.

7. DHYANA (MEDITATION)

Meditation is the sweet bliss of connecting to oneness and to the true self. Where dharana is the emphasis on focus, dhyana is the release of focus and the fluid exploration and experience of awareness. Here, the mind and body experience extreme and blissful peace, and we can begin to understand the true nature of the self and the ever-expansive energy of the infinite universe. Even just a few minutes of dhyana can be deeply rejuvenating and healing.

8. SAMADHI (UNION WITH THE LIFE FORCE)

You've "made" it! Samadhi is freedom from illusion, union with oneness, and pure consciousness. This is the merging of humanity with ecstasy. This is the ultimate "goal" of yoga as a whole: it's where life force flows, love is the default, and fear is nonexistent. This is soul magic: oneness with the divine. The ability to live from this space and integrate it into daily, modern life is where true self-mastery happens. This, of course, has a ripple effect on all of humanity and the planet.

Learning to be in our bodies is a huge benefit of a yoga practice. In our modern world, so many of us live in our heads—we live from the neck up, in our intellect. We forget we have a body and that we have to treat it with reverence. We have taught ourselves to ignore or overrule what our bodies are telling us—that it needs to eat, rest, stretch, and be listened to. A large part of my teaching is helping students become embodied, or come back to their bodies.

—*Dan,* YOGA TEACHER

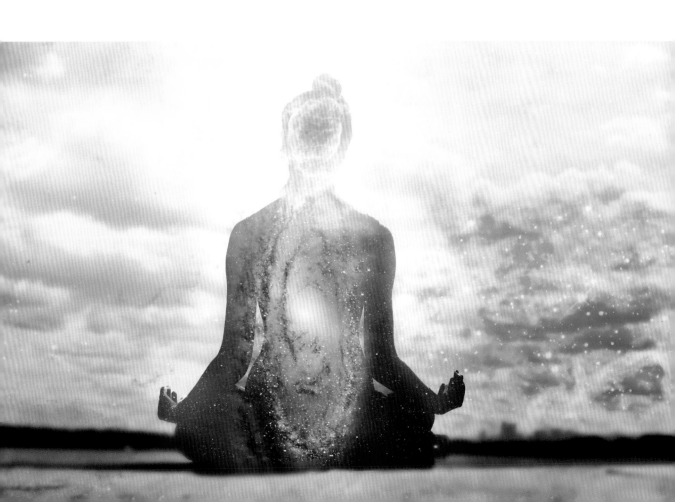

Which Type of Yoga Is Right for You?

———— • ————

Exploring the timeless dimension of the eight limbs of yoga allows you to truly *embody* the original and ancient intention of yoga. But we also live in the modern world, and in this time and place, yoga has a different focus. There are many different asanas that are labeled "yoga"; they were developed long after *The Yoga Sutras* was written and have evolved along with the world. They are all healing. They are all physical. And they all have the potential to help you connect more with your inner self—or at the very least break a sweat. Different types of asana will resonate with different people depending on both the desired level of exertion and the desired level of inward travel.

HATHA

Hatha means "force" and relates to anything that involves physical movement. Modern yoga as we know it today stems from this root. Hatha is typically slow, deep, and gentle movement. It stretches the body, relaxes the mind, and directs attention inward. Hatha yoga is perfect if you're just beginning your yoga journey or if you need to wind down after a hard day or a strenuous workout.

ASHTANGA

Ashtanga yoga is defined by rigidity and a set sequence. This form of yoga focuses on training the mind and body to perform outside of the norm, with a challenging physical practice that directs the dharana (or focus) on the sequence of a moving meditation. If you are a serious athlete or love a good physical and regimented challenge, this might be the yoga path for you.

VINYASA

While Ashtanga promotes rigidity, Vinyasa represents the other side of the coin, with a focus on fluidity and flow. The sequences of movement are aligned with the breath for harmonious coordination. Adapted from Ashtanga in the 1980s, Vinyasa is the most popular class you'll find at your local yoga studio. If you enjoy dance, ballet, or other forms of expressive movement, vinyasa yoga might be a good choice for you.

KUNDALINI

Kundalini yoga focuses on the nervous system and awakening the masculine and feminine energies within all of us, helping that energy ascend from the root chakra (base of the spine) to the crown chakra (above the top of head). This form of yoga was also referred to in the *Vedas* and was a science of energy and spiritual philosophy before it was a physical practice. It is extremely powerful and transformative. If you are fascinated by the chakras or want to explore moving energy throughout your body, Kundalini yoga might be perfect for you.

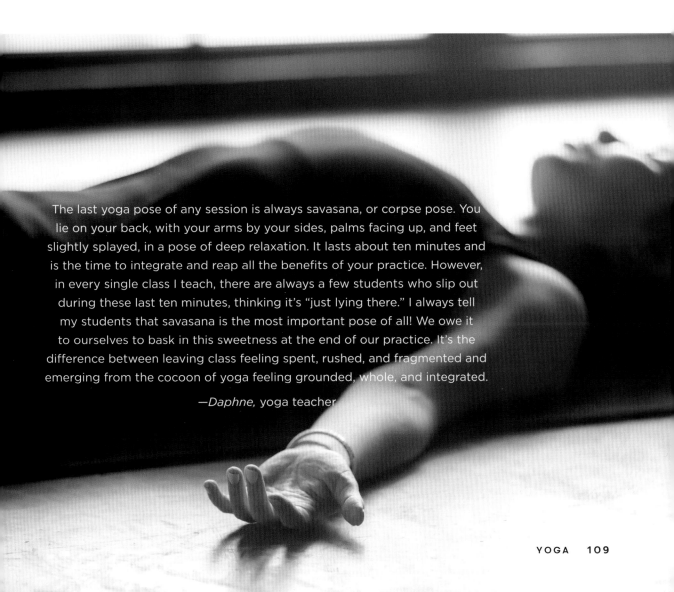

The last yoga pose of any session is always savasana, or corpse pose. You lie on your back, with your arms by your sides, palms facing up, and feet slightly splayed, in a pose of deep relaxation. It lasts about ten minutes and is the time to integrate and reap all the benefits of your practice. However, in every single class I teach, there are always a few students who slip out during these last ten minutes, thinking it's "just lying there." I always tell my students that savasana is the most important pose of all! We owe it to ourselves to bask in this sweetness at the end of our practice. It's the difference between leaving class feeling spent, rushed, and fragmented and emerging from the cocoon of yoga feeling grounded, whole, and integrated.

—*Daphne*, yoga teacher

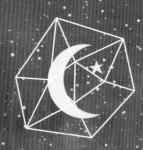

PART 3

COSMIC MAGIC

We are all born equipped to communicate "beyond the veil." Everything from mediumship to tarot is a tool for divine communion with the entire cosmos, and it's here that we can gain guidance from something bigger than ourselves—or perhaps we should call it the biggest part of ourselves. We are never alone in life, even when we feel broken, downtrodden, and abandoned. We all have spirit guides, angels, ancestors, and animal messengers who are waiting for us to make a connection with them. We aren't meant to go it alone, and our soul reaches out to make sure that we never do.

We are spiritual beings who have chosen to undergo a human experience. *Choice* is the key word, and once we understand this, we can better grasp the *why* behind events in our lives that seem to be cruel and unusual punishment. Through past life regression and mediumship, we can begin to understand not only that we carry lessons from one life to another, but also that we never really die. Energy cannot be created or destroyed; therefore, the bodies that we walk around in here on the Earth are only one iteration of the thousands of facets of our soul.

Cosmic magic is all that can be felt but isn't (typically) physically seen. And it's in the evolution of our spirit that we can level up in our next life and move into a new, more divinely aligned existence. Much of this is done in the three-dimensional world through astrology, meditation, shadow work, spirit communication, and the deep healing that comes from past life regression.

ASTROLOGY

"We're made of star stuff."

—*Carl Sagan*

Do you love to check out your horoscope in the newspaper? Yes, well, this chapter is not that. Astrology is more than your sun-sign horoscope, written in such a way that it could apply to just about anyone (even though they're fun to read!).

Almost every ancient civilization invented and subscribed to their own type of astrology. How could they not, when stargazing was the best nightly entertainment around? Their eyes and hearts were filled each night with glittering, shining, bright light that was so magnificent and mysterious that entire civilizations lived by the movements of the planets, stars, and moon. The ancients learned what science now proves: the movements in the night sky correspond to the seasons, the tides, the harvest, and our bodies (read: everything!), so it's no wonder the entire world was, and still is, deeply captivated by the light from the heavens.

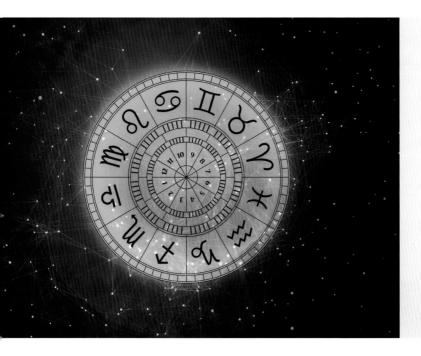

"The starry vault of heaven is in truth the open book of cosmic projection."

—*Carl Jung*

The ancient art of astrology is a favorite divination tool of the modern mystic. In the West, we practice Western astrology, which is based on the alignment of constellations to the tropic of Cancer and the tropic of Capricorn. The birthplace of Western astrology is also the cradle of modern-day civilization: Babylon in Mesopotamia, which is modern-day Iraq. The Mesopotamians left behind the most meticulous surviving records of the genesis of astrology. They methodically mapped the sun, moon, planets, and stars. Charting twelve new moons over the course of a solar year, they built the twelve zodiac signs based on the path of the sun across the sky.

There are many moving parts to astrology, more than we could ever cover in one chapter. Here are the main aspects that we love to follow on the regular!

Zodiac Signs, Ruling Planets, and Elements

The twelve zodiac signs we follow in Western astrology are better known today as the sun signs. Your sun sign is the zodiac constellation that the sun was in the moment you were born. Each zodiac sign has a ruling planet, an element, and a mythological symbol, and it corresponds to various parts of the body. Each zodiac sign is also one of three qualities: cardinal, fixed, or mutable.

CARDINAL: Aligned with the start of each season, cardinal signs are the leaders and starters of the zodiac with a self-initiatory spirit.

FIXED: Aligned with the midpoint of each season, fixed signs are able to dig in and hold steady to achieve a goal in routine, work ethic, and relationship.

MUTABLE: Aligned with the end of each season, mutable signs are flexible and adaptable.

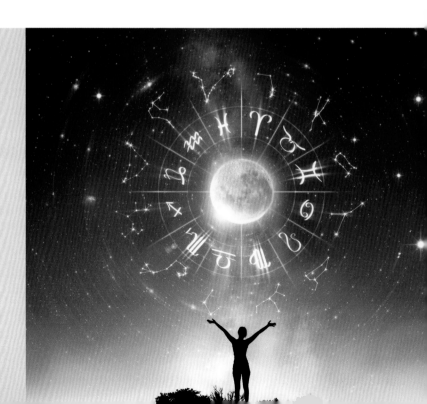

"Astrology is a language. If you understand this language, the sky speaks to you."
—*Dane Rudhyar*

The zodiac starts with Aries at the vernal equinox on March 21, which marks the beginning of spring and the astrological new year. Many consider the astrological new year to be much more of a "new beginning" than January 1 on the Gregorian calendar. Aries is a fire sign, so the zodiac calendar begins with fire and then unfolds sequentially with earth, air, water, and fire again, through all twelve signs.

ARIES

RULING PLANET: Mars, The God of War

ELEMENT: Fire

SYMBOL: The Ram

BODY PARTS: Head, brain, eyes

QUALITY: Cardinal

TRAITS: Aries is the leader of the zodiac. Not only because it's the first sign, but because the fiery ram takes charge, leads the pack, and is very driven. Aries is all action, impulsivity, and a quickness to react.

TAURUS

RULING PLANET: Venus, The Goddess of Love and Pleasure

ELEMENT: Earth

SYMBOL: The Bull

BODY PARTS: Ear, neck, throat

QUALITY: Fixed

TRAITS: Taurus is the first earth sign of the zodiac and is very in touch with the sensual and the material. Slow, steady, and naturally abundant, Taurus truly indulges the senses and understands the value of wealth creation.

GEMINI

RULING PLANET: Mercury, The God of Communication

ELEMENT: Air

SYMBOL: The Twins

BODY PARTS: Lungs, arms, hands

QUALITY: Mutable

TRAITS: Gemini is the only sign in the zodiac represented by human form, and moreover by two of them. This busy, talkative, social, and cerebral air sign is a master communicator. Learning is of utmost importance to Gemini, and sharing that learning with others is incredibly fulfilling.

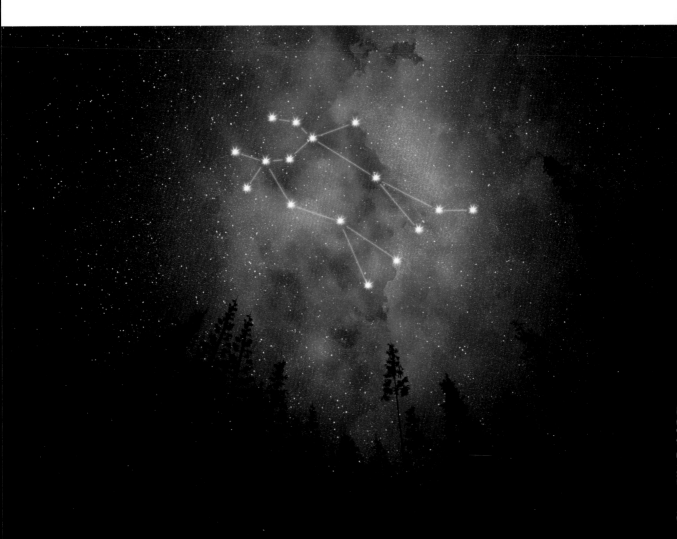

CANCER

RULING PLANET: The Moon (technically a luminary, not a planet), Goddess of the Divine Feminine

ELEMENT: Water

SYMBOL: The Crab

BODY PARTS: Stomach, breasts

QUALITY: Cardinal

TRAITS: Cancer is the goddess of the home and family. Ruled by the moon and pulled with the tides, this crab is soft and vulnerable on the inside with a hard home of a shell. Cancer is the embodiment of the divine feminine and the mother figure. We are reminded of unconditional love from Cancer.

LEO

RULING PLANET: The Sun (technically a luminary, not a planet), God of Light

ELEMENT: Fire

SYMBOL: The Lion

BODY PARTS: Heart, spine

QUALITY: Fixed

TRAITS: Leo is ruled by the sun and, similarly, most certainly loves to be the center of attention and the universe. This vibrant, kind, loving lion reminds us all to shine our light and to be unapologetic about opening our hearts.

VIRGO

RULING PLANET: Mercury, The God of Communication

ELEMENT: Earth

SYMBOL: The Maiden

BODY PARTS: Small intestine, pancreas, liver

QUALITY: Mutable

TRAITS: Virgo is the most thoughtful, logical, and organized sign in the zodiac. This health-conscious earth sign will work to solve everyone's problems while reminding us all that health is the epicenter of life and that structure is soothing.

LIBRA

RULING PLANET: Venus, The Goddess of Love and Pleasure

ELEMENT: Air

SYMBOL: The Scales

BODY PARTS: Kidneys, endocrine system

QUALITY: Cardinal

TRAITS: Libra, ruled by Venus, loves beauty, design, art, romance, and relationships. This Earth sign is all about the beauty around us and how we can benefit from recognizing the love that also lies within. Represented by the scales, Libra is also weighing one option against another and seeks balance.

SCORPIO

RULING PLANET: Pluto, The God of the Underworld

ELEMENT: Water

SYMBOL: The Scorpion

BODY PARTS: Genitals, large intestine

QUALITY: Fixed

TRAITS: Scorpio is the deep, shadowy, sensual, powerful scorpion that is not afraid of the dark. Armed with a stinger, Scorpio is quick to react and kill its "prey," but it is also an incredibly sensual and magnificent creature.

SAGITTARIUS

RULING PLANET: Jupiter, The King of the Gods and The God of Sky and Thunder

ELEMENT: Fire

SYMBOL: The Archer

BODY PARTS: Hips, thighs, circulation

QUALITY: Mutable

TRAITS: Sagittarius is the adventure junkie of the zodiac, always looking for the next national or international thrill. Sagittarians have big ideas, love to study, and indulge in all that life has to offer. Sagittarius has the gift of perspective.

CAPRICORN

RULING PLANET: Saturn, The God of Structure

ELEMENT: Earth

SYMBOL: The Sea Goat

BODY PARTS: Knees, skeleton, teeth

QUALITY: Cardinal

TRAITS: Capricorn is the pragmatic and structured sign of the zodiac we all need in our lives to keep us on track. Ruled by Saturn, these CEOs of the zodiac thrive with order and are incredibly goal driven, but they also understand the benefits of the adage "work hard, play hard."

AQUARIUS

RULING PLANET: Uranus, The God of the Sky

ELEMENT: Air

SYMBOL: The Water Bearer

BODY PARTS: Nervous system

QUALITY: Fixed

TRAITS: Aquarius is the nonconforming humanitarian of the zodiac who will be the first to stand against injustice and to hold a picket sign at a rally. Those born in this sign are the ones who fight for the future and are never afraid to let their freak flag fly.

PISCES

RULING PLANET: Neptune, The God of the Sea

ELEMENT: Water

SYMBOL: The Two Fish

BODY PARTS: Feet, lymphatic system

QUALITY: Mutable

TRAITS: Pisces is by far the most mystical sign in the zodiac. Represented by two fish, Pisces is a sign of duality and otherworldly ways of life. Always thinking magically, Pisces is truly a magical creature.

"The soul of the newly born baby is marked for life by the pattern of the stars at the moment it comes into the world, unconsciously remembers it, and remains sensitive to the return of configurations of a similar kind."

—*Johannes Kepler*

There's More to Astrology Than That!

The average person tends to think of astrology as merely a sun-sign horoscope, but it is much more than that. Beyond the sun sign, there are various planetary aspects that come together "like a symphony," as astrologer Colin Bedell so eloquently described in his book, *A Little Bit of Astrology*. Every individual part affects the whole and, in turn, how we look at our inner and outer worlds.

Natal Charts

Also known as a birth chart, a natal chart is a snapshot of the exact moment you took your first breath on Earth. A natal chart encompasses all planets, houses, nodes, asteroids, and aspects in one beautiful and foretelling graph. To create a natal chart, you'll need your exact birth date, time, and location (if you don't have that, an astrologer can help to decipher important aspects of your chart).

Your natal chart is your cosmic fingerprint that is unique to you. It's a blueprint of your personality and life trajectory. Great insight and wisdom can be gained from analyzing your chart and by looking at the house placement and relation of all planets to each other. An astrology reading with a seasoned astrologer is akin to, and sometimes more insightful than, a therapy session, as the astrologer peers into the makeup of your soul in this lifetime and shares helpful tools to offer support and guidance along your soul's path. Understanding your unique natal chart is one of the best self-awareness tools for the modern mystic.

MOON SIGN

While the sun sign gets a lot of play in Western astrology, your moon sign is a critical, truth-telling aspect of your natal chart. Your moon sign is found by determining what zodiac sign the moon was in when you were born. The moon passes through each sign roughly every two days, and it rules our emotions and how we engage in relationship with ourselves. The moon placement in your chart reveals "the inner you." This is the part of yourself that only *you* know the full depth of. The sign the moon was in when you were born will govern your deepest soul needs and wants at a subconscious level, thus understanding your specific "moon sign" placement is critical to the spiritual seeker.

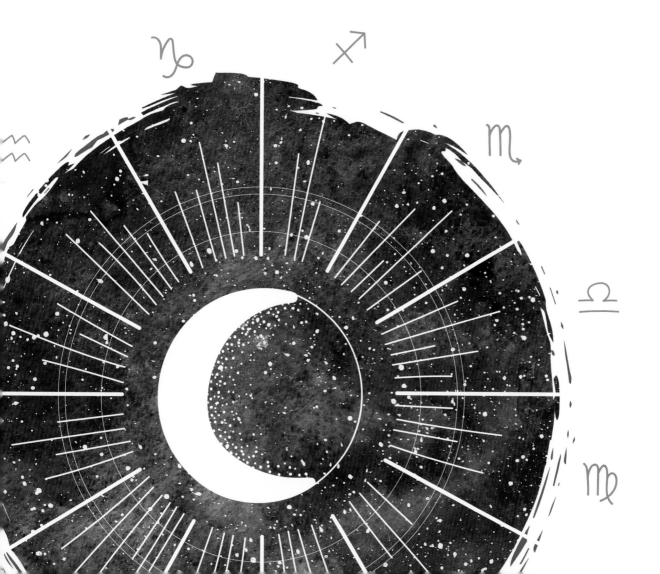

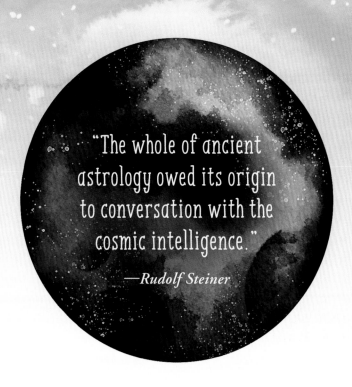

"The whole of ancient astrology owed its origin to conversation with the cosmic intelligence."

—*Rudolf Steiner*

RISING SIGN

Your rising sign, also known as your ascendant, is the zodiac sign that was rising over the eastern horizon at the time of your birth. This placement determines the way that others see you and the first impression you make. It can be thought of as the way you express yourself outwardly via your physical appearance and outward-facing personality and emotions, although this might not be your true nature at the core. It's the outer layer of a multilayered, complex being. For example, if your rising sign is Scorpio and your sun sign is Leo, you may be initially perceived as someone with more Scorpio personality traits (a quiet, mysterious observer) than a flamboyant, attention-seeking Leo.

Phases of the Moon

Like everything in nature, the moon is constantly changing and is always in motion. Forever flowing between darkness and light, the phases of the moon are one of the most ancient ways to track time and the rhythms of nature.

The moon not only pulls the tides, it also pulls on us! We are made up of 70 to 80 percent water, and we are affected by the moon depending on the phase it's in. The moon moves through eight distinct phases, with every degree of movement affecting us.

The new moon is the beginning of the cycle, and as the moon moves through its phases, its light increases—this is called waxing. The moonlight increases until the full moon, and then immediately the light recedes again, which is called waning.

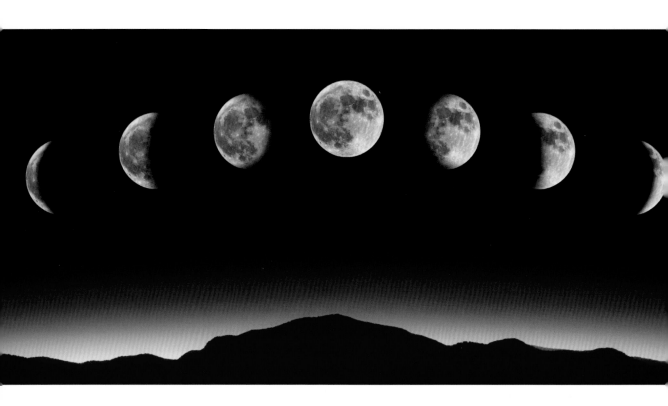

phases of the moon is a magnificent way to connect your desires with the rhythm of nature. This is also a beautiful way to understand the cycle that desires and manifestations must undergo in order to be fully realized to their greatest potential. Below are the implications of each phase.

NORTH AND SOUTH LUNAR NODES

New Moon	A time to plant literal and figurative seeds to set intentions for new beginnings and manifestation cycles
Waxing Crescent Moon	Pure potential and the increase of light and movement
First Quarter Half Moon	Action and commitment are strong while momentum builds
Waxing Gibbous Moon	Practice patience and edit desires as necessary
Full Moon	A time to release, realign, shed, and illuminate what was once in darkness
Waning Gibbous Moon	Practice gratitude and acceptance, go within and explore core changes
Third Quarter Half Moon	A time to give back, adjust as you go, and release what's unnecessary
Waning Crescent Moon	Reflect on the journey, rest, recharge, restore, and surrender

The lunar nodes are mathematical points in the sky, and the north and south nodes in your chart always fall in opposite zodiac signs. So, if you have an Aries north node, then your south node is Libra, and vice versa. The nodes are seldom discussed in a mainstream way, but they are important because they are linked to your life purpose and customized self-mastery, as well as to what you have already mastered in past lives. The north node represents your karmic path and the lessons you are here to learn. The south node reveals the challenges and gifts you bring in from previous lifetimes (see the chapter on past life regression).

When you determine your north and south node placements, it is like discovering a north star on your path to your life's purpose. You might note that the north node placement signifies traits and activities that do not come easily to you. You will relate far more to your south node traits—we all do. Over the course of your lifetime, you will journey more toward developing the north node traits, and then eventually learn to balance the south node traits you are inherently good at with the north node traits you must master through discipline.

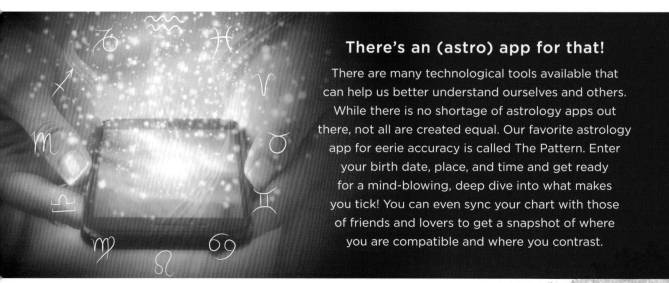

There's an (astro) app for that!

There are many technological tools available that can help us better understand ourselves and others. While there is no shortage of astrology apps out there, not all are created equal. Our favorite astrology app for eerie accuracy is called The Pattern. Enter your birth date, place, and time and get ready for a mind-blowing, deep dive into what makes you tick! You can even sync your chart with those of friends and lovers to get a snapshot of where you are compatible and where you contrast.

MEDITATION

"If you are quiet enough, you will hear the flow of the universe. You will feel its rhythm. Go with this flow. Happiness lies ahead. Meditation is key."

—*Buddha*

It is a paradox that often the people who find it hardest to slow their racing thoughts and to tune in to their inner life need meditation the most. All those calm, centered meditation gurus who seem to never break a sweat? They were once just like all the rest of us—until they found meditation.

It's no secret that so many people swear by meditation for the very simple fact that *it helps people feel better!* Overall, meditation is said to be a boon for happiness, productivity, and creativity, as well as the most effective way to commune with the divine. In addition to producing that natural high we knew as children but have since misplaced—the one that comes from living in the moment—meditation is a salve for many "diseases" of modernity: stress, anxiety, depression, inflammation in the body, heart disease, and insomnia. Meditation's healing benefits seem to treat the whole person—physiologically, spiritually, emotionally, and mentally—and doctors are even prescribing it for their patients.

Now that science has proven the benefits of meditation, it has been widely incorporated into many Western systems where spiritual practices are otherwise largely missing, including schools, corporations, prisons, and even the Marine Corps. It is roughly estimated that up to 500 million people regularly practice meditation all over the world. If you aren't yet one of those millions, consider becoming one. Apps like Calm, Insight Timer, and many more now make meditation simple and convenient. Because, oddly, in our fast-paced world, sitting quietly and reflecting are something we just do not have time for!

The Short History of a Long-time Practice

Like many of the ancient healing techniques discussed in this book, the precise beginnings of meditation are impossible to pin down. However, archeologists agree that this transformative practice began around 5000 to 3500 BCE, and thus dates back further than civilized society.

Although meditation can be found in ancient religious texts the world over, the practice as a ritual ingredient of a spiritual path is most closely associated with Buddhism, as it was Siddhārtha Gautama, otherwise known as the Buddha, who really ignited this ancient healing modality. The Buddha lived in Southeast Asia some 2,600 years ago, and he remains the greatest meditation guru ever.

Meditation was largely unknown outside Asia until the 18th century, when ancient yoga texts finally made their way to scholars in the Western world. In 1958, literary folk hero Jack Kerouac published *Dharma Bums*, which attracted people in droves to Eastern spirituality and meditation. Hatha yoga and transcendental meditation began gaining popularity in the 1960s, and today, *meditation* is a household word.

"Meditation is a process of lightening up, of trusting the basic goodness of what we have and who we are, and of realizing that any wisdom that exists, exists in what we already have."

—*Pema Chödrön,* THE WISDOM OF NO ESCAPE

The Buddha Effect

According to Buddha, meditation is an imperative practice on the road to enlightenment and true happiness—a state of being for which every human longs. The path that the Buddha taught is considered the "Golden Mean" because it illuminates the idea that there is no need to go to any extreme on a spiritual path, neither in indulgence nor in abstinence.

The Buddha's central teaching is that the mind is the core and determiner of our existence. Mind is dual. Meditation helps us transform our thoughts from evil to good, dark to light, negative to positive. A similar idea in Hindu tradition holds that the human mind is equipped with the creative potency of God. You are the sum of your thoughts and desires, not only of this life but also of your past lives. You co-create your life with God via your mental activity. Thus, you become what you think. Meditation stills your subconscious, muddled thoughts and redirects them to a more elevated place.

"Meditation brings wisdom; lack of meditation leaves ignorance."

—*The Buddha*

Which Type of Meditation Is Right for You?

————— • —————

There are countless ways to meditate, and ultimately it is, like anything else, a customizable experience where you find what works best *for you*. Below are some of our favorite types of meditation to get you started.

VEDIC MEDITATION

The oldest documented form of meditation, this is the technique from which all other meditation techniques derive. Using a mantra, or repetitive sound, the mind begins to settle down and focus on the vibration of that sound, turning away from the "monkey mind" thoughts that otherwise stream unencumbered through our minds. There is no need to try to "empty" the mind here, as it's all about *distracting* the mind. By repeating one word or sound over and over, your mind is occupied and stops dwelling on all the other stressful and detrimental things coursing through your headspace. Worry, fear, and anxiety all get pushed aside. The goal is to disrupt the everyday thoughts that run on autopilot, because they tend to be frantic and unkind. See the section on manifestation (page 56) for more about the power of rewiring your subconscious mind to true healing. Meditation is also a powerful tool in that reconditioning process.

Vedic meditation has four major benefits: it reduces stress and anxiety, it improves heart health, it improves sleep quality, and it unleashes creativity. If you are struggling in one of these areas—for example, you experience insomnia, have cardiovascular issues, or are facing a creative block—then vedic meditation may be for you.

VIPASSANA MEDITATION

Vipassana means "insight" and "to see things as they really are." Vipassana meditation is a type of mindfulness meditation that originated in the Buddhist tradition, and it is said that Vipassana is an unbroken lineage, meaning it has been handed down from teacher to student continuously for millennia, directly from the Buddha. Through mindfulness, watching the breath, and self-observation, we can notice our thoughts and physical sensations, without judgment or attachment. In this way, we gain insight into the true nature of reality: impermanence, suffering, and non-self. We come to understand that everything is impermanent: our thoughts, our sensations, ourselves. When we delude ourselves about the nature of reality, we experience suffering. And when we understand that there is no unchanging, permanent self, we enter a state of bliss and compassion.

This sacredly preserved method cannot be learned via YouTube or a weekend workshop. A ten-day residential course is required to properly learn Vipassana meditation, during which you can expect to undergo rigorous spiritual work. But if you struggle with being judgmental, jealous, or fearful, this form of meditation may be very helpful for you.

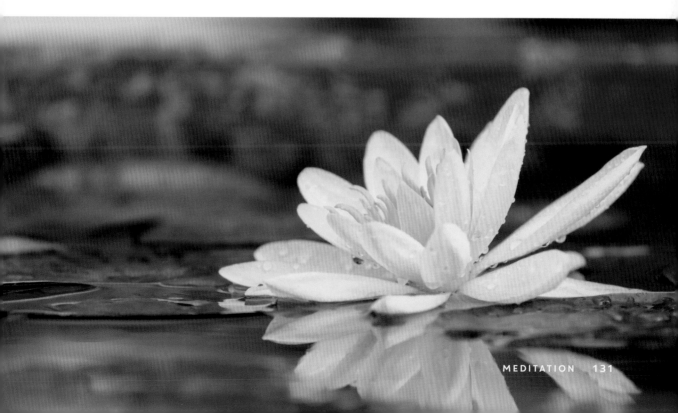

"With every breath, the old moment is lost; a new moment arrives. We exhale and we let go of the old moment. It is lost to us. In doing so, we let go of the person we used to be. We inhale and breathe in the moment that is becoming. In doing so, we welcome the person we are becoming. We repeat the process. This is meditation. This is renewal. This is life."

—Lama Surya Das,
LETTING GO OF THE PERSON YOU USED TO BE

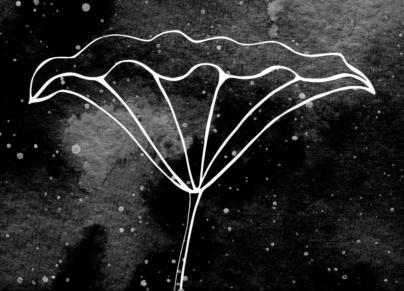

MANTRA MEDITATION

The Sanskrit word *mantra* means "a tool for the mind" on the path to enlightenment and pure happiness. In the traditional form, a mantra is a one-syllable sound that probably doesn't even have a literal translation, such as "om." It's more about the vibration of the sound and the way the tongue hits the roof of the mouth. However, today mantras have been extended to include positive affirmations, such as "I am whole. I am healthy. I am complete."

We can think about only one thing at a time, and mantras can hijack our usual, sometimes judgmental or negative line of thought with a focus on one sound vibration or positive thought, keeping us in the present moment. Staying in the present moment is, after all, the one and only entry point to connecting with the world of divine spirit.

People use mantra meditation to cope with fears, to invite sleep, to clear their chakras (see page 33), to assist with visualization (see page 65) and with sound healing (see page 142), and to transform consciousness. If you want to build mental toughness, boost motivation, kick a bad habit, or uproot deep-seated negativity, mantra meditation may be helpful for you.

LOVING-KINDNESS MEDITATION

The loving-kindness meditation style aims to cultivate compassion through softening your heart and mind through kind thoughts and intentionally loving phrases. It's essentially a mantra-based technique but the purpose is to create love and peace for all sentient beings on the planet.

Once in a comfortable position, begin saying these phrases silently in your mind: *May I be happy. May I be healthy. May I be safe from harm. May I live with peace and ease.* Once you meditate on those phrases for yourself, then think of someone you love and replace "I" with their name. Eventually you can do this meditation for "the world" or "all sentient beings." You can also do this meditation for someone with whom you have conflict or harbor feelings of anger, fear, or jealousy. Simply replace "I" with their name. This is often the hardest meditation for people to do, but it is an amazingly transformational tool for forgiveness.

If you struggle with self-love, anger toward another person, or concern and anxiety for the state of the world, loving-kindness meditation, which cultivates compassion, may be perfect for you.

Even though my father had passed years ago, I was still angry with him and blamed him for the problems in my life and in my relationships. My therapist suggested I try loving-kindness meditation, and he guided me through it. I came to understand that he did the best he could, that he had suffered too, and that we are all human. Through this meditation, something in my heart shifted, and I was able to heal my anger and find forgiveness.

—*Erik, 34*

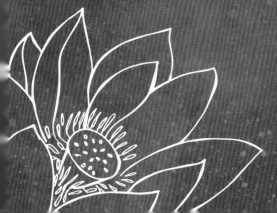

ZEN MEDITATION

We've all heard the word *Zen*, but what does it mean? An ancient Buddhist tradition, Zen meditation, also known as Zazen, was, like Vipassana, taught by the Buddha. This minimalist-style meditation technique does not include arduous mantras or rigid instructions. All it takes is getting into one of the correct postures (see step 2 on the next page), placing your left hand on top of your right, both palm-up, thumbs touching, just in front of your navel, taking a deep breath, and then quietly chilling. And what about the inevitable thoughts that arise? Simply allow them; watch them come and go like passing clouds and bring your attention back to your breath and your posture. Some people find it intimidating to have no real rules or anchor during meditation, but for others it's the only way. We say give everything a try once and see what works best, as always, *for you*.

Zen meditation is all about emptying the mind; after consistent practice, your mind will learn to settle down naturally. If you struggle with maintaining attention and focus, Zen meditation may be helpful for you.

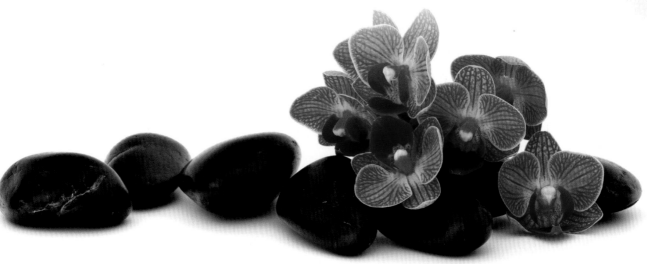

How to Meditate

Although meditation is quite simple, that doesn't mean it is easy. Here are a few steps that will help you slip into, and maintain, a meditative state more smoothly.

1. Select the type of meditation style you want to follow (refer to the previous pages or research online if one of these doesn't resonate with you).

2. Some people meditate while lying down, kneeling, or seated with legs crossed or uncrossed. If you're kneeling or in a seated position, be sure to sit up straight and align your spine. Imagine a string in the center of your crown lifting you like a marionette.

3. Let your belly be soft. We have been taught to suck in our belly and tighten our core so our natural bulges don't show. But for meditation, you want your belly to be soft and relaxed, so that your breath can deepen. Think of your belly like a balloon that fills with air and empties, expanding and contracting with ease.

4. Many people find it helpful to focus on their nostrils, feeling the breath enter and exit from the tip of their nose. Follow the breath going all the way down to the bottom of your lungs and drifting up and out again. See the sidebar on breathwork for more information.

5. Bring your attention to your mantra, your breath, or another point of focus. Some people like to gaze softly at a candle flame or a sacred object.

6. Whenever you notice your mind wandering—and it will—simply bring it back to your point of focus. Do not get frustrated with your wandering mind. The mind's job is to think, and it takes a great deal of practice to teach it to let go of thought for even just a few moments.

7. Rest in this space of nonjudgmental awareness, bringing your mind back to your point of focus again and again.

8. When you are done, let out a long, slow breath, emptying your lungs of all air. Relax for a few minutes and begin to breathe more naturally. Thank yourself for making this time for your practice, and rest in a sense of gratitude for the calm and peace meditation brings you.

9. Allow your eyes to open slowly and adjust to your surroundings. Wiggle your fingers and toes to wake them up, then shake out your arms and legs if you need to. Slowly stand up. You might feel a bit dizzy from all the oxygen reaching your brain, so give yourself time to acclimate and don't just jump up when you're done.

10. Try to bring the sensations and feelings of calmness with you as you go about your day.

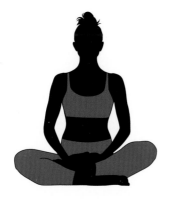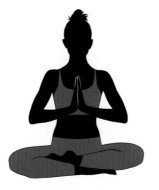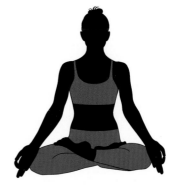

How to Create a Meditation Practice

No matter which meditation path resonates with you, all of them can add value and healing to your life. The key is commitment, and regular practice is essential. Meditating in the morning and evening before bed is most effective, even if it's for only a few minutes at first. As your practice strengthens, aim for 20 minutes in the morning and 20 minutes in the evening. Some people set a timer so they don't have to wonder (or think about) the length of their meditation time. Don't meditate lying down or in bed; the purpose is not to fall asleep, and if you are too comfortable or meditating right before bed, you could drift off into dreamland.

No two meditation sessions are alike, so don't compare them to each other. Some days you will find it hard to settle and other days meditation will just flow. You might want to keep a journal to document changes you experience in your life, insights you might have during meditation, or methods that work for you. This journal can keep you motivated to maintain a consistent practice, especially on days when meditating is the last thing you want to do (and those are the days when you definitely need it!). The effects of meditation are cumulative and subtle, but they are transformative.

"Mindfulness practice means that we commit fully in each moment to be present; inviting ourselves to interface with this moment in full awareness, with the intention to embody as best we can an orientation of calmness, mindfulness, and equanimity right here and right now."

—*Jon Kabat-Zinn*, WHEREVER YOU GO, THERE YOU ARE

Guided Meditation

Let's get one thing clear: meditation is *not* easy. If it were easy to still our minds of our mental chatter, we wouldn't even need something like meditation in the first place. Getting to that place of mental calmness, especially in such a frenzied society, takes practice—and lots of it. Guided meditations are one way to help you sink faster and deeper into a place of stillness.

There are many guided meditations available via YouTube of course, plus apps that offer thousands of guided meditations for everyday use. We highly recommend, however, attending a guided meditation session with other live beating hearts in the room. Why? Besides setting the stage for you to socialize with like-minded people, everything is better when shared, including meditation. When cozied up in a room, meditating together, we can get on the same energetic wavelength as others. Recorded EEG results have proven that brain waves synchronize while meditating. When we harmonize our energy in this profound way, we start to understand that we aren't alone, a valuable realization for the isolated modern mystic.

Breathwork

One of the oldest, most powerful self-healing tools we have can be found right under our noses—literally! Not only is it completely free of charge, but mindful breath control is also extremely potent medicine. Studies show that many people use less than 50 percent of their breathing capacity. This is shallow breathing, and it prevents sufficient oxygen from getting to our brain and other cells. "Breathwork," the act of bringing conscious awareness to this subconscious process, uses various controlled breathing techniques.

Most of us spend our days breathing "vertically," taking short, shallow breaths in our upper chests. Healthy breathing, however, is performed "horizontally," with long, expansive, restful breaths reaching all the way to the bottom of the abdomen. Making full use of our lower lung capacity with deep, slow, intentional breathing paves the way for a calm, peaceful mindset. Whatever controlled breathing modality you opt for, try to commit to it at least twice per day. The goal is to retrain your entire way of breathing. With enough practice and commitment, you'll begin breathing more deeply, without ever thinking about it.

"Feelings come and go like clouds in a windy sky. Conscious breathing is my anchor."

—*Thich Nhat Hanh*

TYPES OF BREATHWORK

Yoga masters manipulate the breath in three phases: inhalation, retention, and exhalation. This practice focuses on the pause, the nothingness, between breaths to reduce stress and improve cognition. In another method, you do not hold your breath at any point of time. As soon as your lungs become full, you start exhaling, and whenever they're empty, you start inhaling again. This creates a cyclical breath pattern that is relaxed and gentle and is said to heighten awareness.

Here is a breathing exercise that will leave you feeling refreshed and at peace.

1. Sit up straight in a comfortable position.

2. Close your eyes and begin to breathe in slow and steady through the nose for a count of 4, allowing your abdomen to expand.

3. Hold your breath for a count of 7.

4. Exhale for a count of 8, this time through the mouth.

5. Visualize a person, place, or thing that brings you ecstatic joy (trick: pets and babies are primo for this!).

6. Express gratitude out loud for your chosen person, place, or thing.

7. Repeat this process three times in a row, or until you feel calm.

Though we take it for granted, when we are short of breath, everything else loses importance and we are reminded of the gravity of life. The fact is that when we take breath for granted, we also take life for granted.

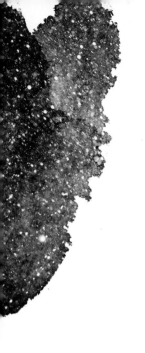

SOUND HEALING

"He who knows the secret of the sound knows the mystery of the whole universe."

—*Hazrat Inayat Khan*

Have you ever listened to music that stirred your soul to the point of tears? Or felt a blue mood transformed by an upbeat, danceable tune? Or stilled a chattering mind with a soothing instrumental track? This is the healing power of sound.

As we touched on in the section on crystal healing (page 24), everything in the universe is vibration, frequency, and energy. Sound travels through the cosmos and through our bodies in the same way—in waves. These waves have been understood across time and cultures to hold immense healing power. From the moment a baby takes its first breath and cries to the moment the last breath of air escapes the lungs before death, we are deeply affected, inspired, and healed by sound. Humans have long used music and song to communicate, celebrate, mourn, and connect. From drums to flutes, rattles to horns, humans have crafted instruments from the surrounding landscape, connecting us even more deeply to the natural world.

The energetic frequency of the mind, body, and soul can be felt up to 5 feet from the body. Because all matter is energy vibrating at different rates, sound can shift the vibration of organs or parts of the body that have gotten out of tune. Every emotion is also associated with a vibration, and by consciously aligning with a specific vibration, we can journey via sound to an emotion we wish to embody. This often happens at a nonverbal, intuitive level that bypasses the thinking brain. In a word, music makes us *feel*.

"Music is the literature of the heart;
it commences where speech ends."

—*Alphonse de Lamartine*

What Is Sound Healing?

Although listening to music is a form of sound healing, sound healing is more than just that. Sound is measured in hertz, the same as our brain waves. Our brain produces chemicals and hormones as well as electricity, so it only makes sense that to impact, heal, and altar brain waves we use sound. Brain waves occur in five distinct states that range from the low frequency akin to a drum to a high vibration akin to a flute:

The Oldest Instrument

Technically, the voice is the oldest instrument, but the first *manmade* instrument dates back more than 40,000 years, when tribes in northern Australia created the didgeridoo, or yidaki. This wooden instrument was made from fallen eucalyptus branches that were hollowed out, either by termites or by hand, and it is thought to be the oldest instrument in human history. The deep bass of the didgeridoo has a low vibration that is in alignment with the root chakra and the earth.

1. DELTA WAVES (0.5 TO 3 HZ)

Delta is the lowest and most penetrating brain wave that we experience in the deepest meditation or dreamless sleep. Delta waves are also the source of our empathy, restoration, and healing.

2. THETA WAVES (3 TO 8 HZ)

Theta waves occur in twilight sleep and are where our learning, memory, and intuition are activated. This frequency draws our attention inward and allows soul exploration and going beyond our conscious awareness.

3. ALPHA WAVES (8 TO 12 HZ)

Alpha is the brain's resting state, where thoughts quietly flow, such as when we are in meditation. In this state we can access calmness, alertness, and the mind–body connection.

4. BETA WAVES (12 TO 38 HZ)

Beta is our normal waking state of consciousness and cognition. This fast frequency helps us solve problems, make decisions, and have focused mental activity.

5. GAMMA WAVES (38 TO 42 HZ)

Gamma is the highest frequency and is our quiet and subtle connection to higher states of being, universal love, and altruism. This is where higher consciousness and spiritual emergence take place.

Sound healing methods directly target these states of frequency to attune our energy and bring about healing.

Which Sound Healing Methods Are Right for You?

You don't have to be a musician or a singer to use sound in a healing way. There are many methods you can try that require no more than a recording or your own voice. Other methods require an instrument, such as a gong or singing bowls, but even these don't need any special knowledge or experience.

BINAURAL BEATS

Using different vibrational tones created electronically, binaural beats are a powerful way to use soundwave therapy to access different parts of the brain to help rewire our brain waves and encourage self-healing. In this form of therapy, the right and left ears listen to slightly different frequency tones that are perceived as one. Binaural beats can easily be found on YouTube in all ranges that are aligned to our various moods, chakras, outcomes, goals, and states of being. For example, if you're trying to relax and fall asleep, you'll want to listen to something in the delta or theta range.

Binaural beats have been found to help heal very specific ailments, including PTSD, anxiety, depression, and chronic pain, and they can encourage a deeper connection to our spirituality. If you struggle with one of the ailments listed, binaural beats might be a great sound healing method for you. They are also an excellent way for beginners to get into sound healing, because you don't need to do anything except listen. For best results using binaural beats therapy, practice listening for 15 to 30 minutes every day for 30 to 45 days.

SOUND HEALING AND THE CHAKRAS

Every chakra and internal organ is linked to a primordial hum. (See the chapter on crystal healing for more on the chakras and energy.) The lowest vibration is at the root chakra and the highest is at the crown chakra. By chanting the sound associated with each chakra, we can tune and align the chakras, bringing the entire energetic system into balance. If you are fascinated by the chakra system and want to explore balancing your energy centers, then this type of sound healing might be for you.

CHAKRA	LOCATION	SPIRITUAL QUALITIES	SOUND
Root	Base of your spine	Safety, grounding, protection	LAAM
Sacral	A few inches below your belly button	Integrity, identity, control	VAAM
Solar plexus	Bottom of your sternum	Self-esteem, courage, maturity	RAAM
Heart	Center of your chest	Love, compassion, balance	YAAM
Throat	Over your Adam's apple	Truth, communication, self-expression	HAAM
Third eye	Center of your forehead	Intuition, psychic ability, relationship with higher self	KSHAAM
Crown	Just above the top of your head	Ethics, values, connection to Spirit	OM

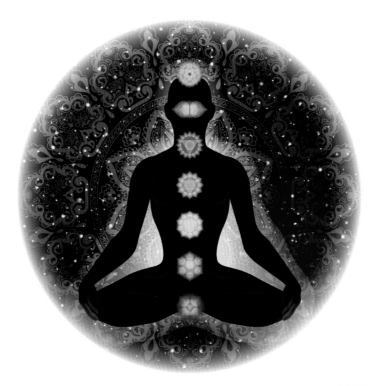

CHANTING

Chanting, or toning, as it is also called, is the harmonization of the human voice to certain frequencies using seven specific vowels. Said to be the primordial sound of the universe and of life, "om" or "aum" is the sound of pure potential. When chanted or hummed, this vibrational frequency is said to bring our soul into harmony with the universe.

We can also chant the sounds of the chakras (see above), ancient spiritual texts, vowels, and prayers. Chanting alone is beneficial, but chanting in a group is extremely powerful. When the intention of the collective is focused, it is like a laser beam that spans space and time, amplifying your vibration exponentially. Chanting reduces fear and anxiety, improves mood, and heals emotional pain.

You don't need to be able to sing or even carry a tune in order to chant, but if you enjoy using your voice as an instrument, then chanting might be a great sound healing method for you to explore.

GONG

The gong is a mystical vehicle of sound and encompasses the entire range of sound that a human ear can hear. This doesn't just stop at the ear, though: sound waves of the gong can be felt through the entire body, down to each individual cell. When metal is struck, electrons become excited and form an electromagnetic field that is palpably felt. It simultaneously affects every chakra and brain wave state. A natural buzz is created in the body as the sound and vibration of the gong are built up and then released. Thus, many mental, physical, emotional, and spiritual ailments can be cleared in gong ceremonies.

Because the gong cuts through mental chatter, it invokes a meditative state and deep relaxation where restoration and healing occur. It aligns the chakras and invigorates the flow of energy through the meridians (energy pathways in the body). It has been found to stimulate the glandular system, soothe the nervous system, and improve sleep.

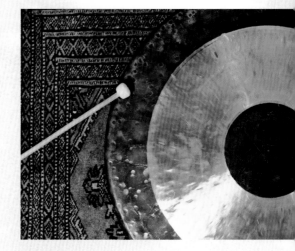

If you love the idea of selecting a special instrument for sound healing, or especially enjoy the gong's resonance, then this sound healing method may be a good fit for you.

> ## "Do you know that our soul is composed of harmony?"
>
> —*Leonardo da Vinci,* NOTEBOOKS

DRUMMING

The sound of the drum mimics the sound of the heartbeat. We are literally born with rhythm, and we are drawn to and calmed by the rhythm of our mother's heartbeat. The anatomy of the drum—a round shape that represents the whole universe—hasn't changed in the thousands and thousands of years that it's been in use.

The resonant sound of the drum can bring raw emotions to the surface and allow you to release them while your mind, which so desperately wants to hold on to pain, is distracted and entranced by repetitive rhythm. Drumming is so ingrained over epochs that even babies have a physical response to the rhythm of the drum.

Drumming has also been shown to lower blood pressure, reduce pain, increase white brain matter, decrease stress, and evoke transcendental experiences. It reconnects us to the heart, and to the source of all life.

You don't need to be a musician to take up drumming; there are drumming classes offered everywhere, such as through adult education programs, yoga studios, and meditation centers. It helps to have a teacher get you started with primal drumming patterns, and you'll get more out of this sound healing method if you practice and stick with it.

SINGING BOWLS

Tibetan brass singing bowls emit pure sonic waves and have been used for thousands of years for meditation and relaxation. Depending on the size of the bowls, they have varying pitches of reverberating tone, plus they make a bell sound when struck directly. You can also find crystal singing bowls that are tuned to each of the main chakras.

The vibrations of singing bowls are so effective because they entrain brain waves to the theta level, a state of deep relaxation, bringing different parts into vibrational alignment. Bowls can be placed on and around the body and played to move stagnant energy and restore balance and vitality.

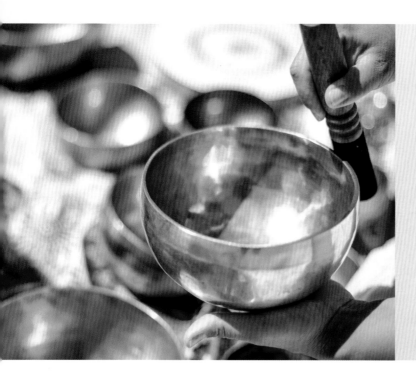

"Music is the mediator between the life of the senses and the life of the spirit."

—*Beethoven*

Singing bowls also balance the chakras, improve energy flow and blood circulation, reduce stress and anxiety, restore spiritual connection, relieve pain, increase mental and emotional clarity, and promote happiness and well-being.

Singing bowls are beautiful objects and come in a range of materials, styles, and tones. It's best to try out various singing bowls in person at a shop so that you can see which resonances you are drawn to and how the reverberating energy affects you.

MUSIC THERAPY

Our hardwired psychological response to music can be measured in day-old infants. Our brains are awakened by the structure, rhythm, and beat of songs. Music therapy can help the brain create new neuropathways to improve learning: that's why children learn the ABCs through song.

Music is the only sensory experience that activates all areas of the brain at the same time. It triggers whole-brain processes and functioning with direct effects on cognitive, emotional, and physical levels. There are two types of music therapy: active (or expressive) music therapy and receptive music therapy. Active music therapy engages people in music making, whether that is singing, playing an instrument, or writing songs. Receptive music therapy involves listening to recorded music, often selected by a music therapist. People can then discuss the feelings the music evokes or what the lyrics mean to them. This type of therapy allows the individual to bypass the thinking, analytical brain and to elicit feelings and mood-states they might not be able to with verbal expression.

Trained music therapists will tell you that music therapy is not about simply plugging in your iPod and listening to music, no matter how moving or relaxing it is. Music therapy has shown evidence-based results in people with Alzheimer's, Parkinson's, autism, aphasia, dementia, and heart disease.

To use music therapy on your own, listen to your intuition and play music that will amplify the state you're in or help you journey to a desired state. As an adjunct to music, you can use guided imagery, progressive muscle relaxation, or other relaxation techniques. Music therapy can also be used in conjunction with singing, dancing, choreography, movement, and art-making to elicit even more powerful responses. And remember: words are spells and lyrics matter, so choose the good ones!

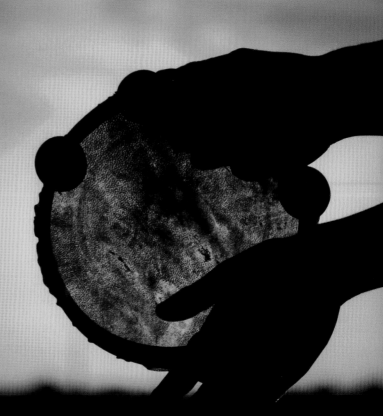

"Man's music is seen as a means of restoring the soul, as well as confused and discordant bodily afflictions, to the harmonic proportions that it shares with the world soul of the cosmos."

—*Plato*

Take a Dip in a Sound Bath

What's a sound bath, you ask?! Well, first, there's no water involved, so leave your swimsuit at home! Sound baths are an ancient form of deep group meditation that consists of an instructor playing various ambient sounds with crystal bowls, singing bowls, drums, chimes, bells, and/or gongs while participants lie on a yoga mat on the floor. The different frequencies of the various sounds draw participants into a deeper meditative state.

An hour-long sound bath can transport you to a place where deep healing can occur, leaving you feeling relaxed and focused, ready to take on the stressors of modern-day life. Sound baths are growing in popularity because they make people feel good, which is the essence of all real healing. A growing number of hospitals are incorporating sound baths as alternative healing options for their patients, and some hospitals are even bringing versions of them to waiting rooms! Visit your local yoga studio or metaphysical outlet—more than likely they have a sound bath scheduled or know where you can find one.

SPIRIT COMMUNICATION

"For every soul, there is a guardian watching it."

—*The Koran*

It is far too easy to feel alone in a modern world that, in many ways, isolates us from each other and increasingly devalues the power of community. Ironically, we are in an age that is more connected than ever on social media, but also more socially secluded than ever on deeper, meaningful, spiritual levels.

However, that we are seemingly "alone" in the three-dimensional world is the greatest illusion from a spiritual vantage point. Each human soul not only has a "guardian" angel watching over it (as expressed in the Koran), but an entire spirit team made up of angels, spirit guides, ancestors, and other divine beings. The team's sole purpose is to guide us to our highest manifestation possible throughout our human life. Therefore, in effect, we are never, ever truly alone.

Many people mistakenly think that only specially gifted "psychics" can communicate with Spirit, but this skill is available to *all*. Like any spiritual technique, spirit communication is a practice, and your ability to listen and receive messages increases with dedication. The more you trust in the communications you receive from the spirit world, rather than write them off as coincidence, the more your spirit team will trust you and send more messages as you heighten your extrasensory perceptions. Therefore, it's important to note that openness and faith are requirements to strengthening your communicative ties to the unseen spirit beings that long to help us on our healing journeys.

Meet Your Spirit Team

Who are we communicating with, exactly? Following are the various entities that spirit communication experts say make up our personalized spirit teams.

ANCESTORS

As discussed in depth in the mediumship chapter (see page 173), people's souls do not die; at death, people merely shed their physical bodies and the soul returns to the ethereal world of spirit. Death is a graduation to another form of life, and our ancestors are still part of our lives after their physical deaths, we just aren't attuned to their vibration. Even so, they still protect us and watch over us.

From the world that lies beyond this human existence, our closest ancestors often become guides and advisors to us from the other side, and when you need guidance, calling on your ancestors will help bring you clarity. This is why ancient and indigenous peoples have always continued to revere their deceased loved ones. Our ancestors never leave us and they can help us as we continue on our earthly life without them here in the physical sense.

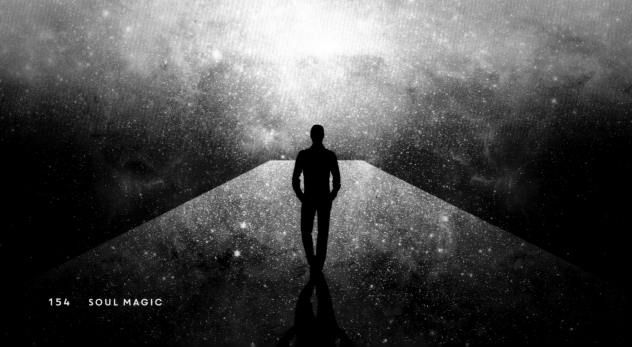

ANGEL GUIDES

Angel communicator and best-selling author Kyle Gray says, "The most beautiful thing about angels is the fact that they are absolutely desperate to help us. When they see us in distress or lost in any way, they're just waiting to be invited to bring the solution." The most important word in this quote is *invited*. Angels are here to help us as guides, but they do not interfere with our free will, so it is vital to invoke angels to guide your life by asking them for help. Make a habit of asking your angels for guidance throughout your day and watch how your life transforms!

> "Angels are so enamored of the language that is spoken in heaven that they will not distort their lips with the hissing and unmusical dialects of men, but speak their own, whether there be any who understand it or not."
>
> —*Ralph Waldo Emerson*

ASCENDED MASTERS

Ascended masters, who were ordinary humans in past incarnations, are spiritually enlightened beings who have gained full union with the divine source. Many ascended masters choose to support and guide people on their own ascension paths and so can join a person's spirit team. Ascended master guidance focuses solely on the ascension process and is of the highest possible vibration. Some of the more well-known ascended masters are Jesus, Buddha, and Confucius.

ELEMENTALS

Also called "nature spirits," elementals include fantastical beings like fairies, mermaids, dragons, elves, gnomes, and more. Nature spirits are the guardians of Mother Earth. Just as humans have guardian angels and spirit guides looking out for us, Mother Earth has elementals who tend to her and help protect her. These nature spirits come to our own spirit teams if we work closely with nature and the protection of our environment. They can also join our teams if we need some play and laughter in our lives, as these spirits love to celebrate and frolic—even to the point of being mischievous!

POWER ANIMALS

Animals can simply be a messenger for a moment of time in your life, as we discuss later in this chapter, or they can be a permanent fixture on your spirit team. Sometimes referred to as "power animals," they offer guidance and protection and help you overcome fear. They can also lend you their specific wisdom and attributes to support you on your journey through life.

And we just know you are asking whether your deceased pet could possibly join your guidance team … and the answer is a resounding yes! Just like our human ancestors, deceased pets can claim a spot on our protective spirit team.

SPIRIT GUIDES

Ancestors and angels have been popular through most of history, but spirit guides are helpers that typically don't get quite as much attention. In the words of world-renowned spiritual medium Susanne Wilson, "Spirit guides are the unsung heroes [of the spiritual world]. They work mainly behind the scenes, giving you gentle nudges along your path." Yet spirit guides are extremely important to us on our journey here on this planet. If you are interested in taking a meditative journey to meet your spirit guides, we recommend the "Guidance Quest: Connect with Your Spirit Guides" meditation available at carefreemedium.com.

"Your spirit guides
and angels will never
let you down as
you build a rapport
with them. In the
end, they may be the
only ones who don't
let you down."

—*Linda Deir*

The Many Voices of Spirit

How can we learn to decipher the heavenly language of our spirit teams
so we can absorb their wisdom? Communication with the spirit world
happens through our various senses. You've likely heard the word *clairvoyance*
and know it relates somehow to "psychic powers" of communicating
with the spirit world, but did you know that clairvoyance is only one
of eight ways to experience messages from the invisible realms?

Some of the best spiritual communicators in the world have each of the eight "clairs" to
some extent; others are strongest in one or two. The important thing is that no matter
what our current abilities, whether we are a master medium or have never yet felt the
presence of spirit communication in our lives, we can learn to develop our innate spirit
communication skills through dedication and practice. Let's look at each of the clair-senses.

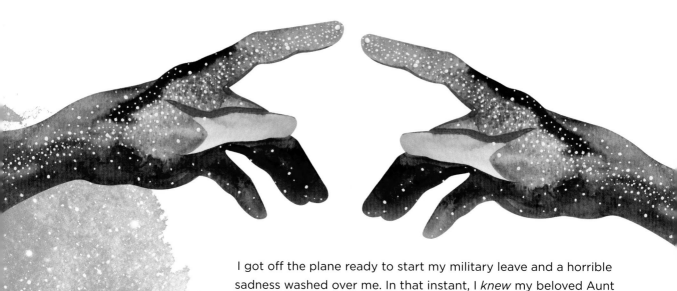

I got off the plane ready to start my military leave and a horrible
sadness washed over me. In that instant, I *knew* my beloved Aunt
Bea had died. I found a pay phone and called her house. My
uncle picked up and I could hear crying in the background. His
voice was strained. Holding back tears, he told me my aunt had
passed about an hour ago. It was uncanny how I simply *knew*.

—*Frank, 68*

CLAIRVOYANCE: CLEAR SEEING

The most popular of the "clairs," clairvoyance means a person sees extrasensory impressions and symbols in the form of visual images in their mind's third eye. Vivid prophetic dreams and visions that flash into a person's mind's eye also indicate clairvoyance. Clairvoyants can see, rather than just sense, entities in the spiritual realms, such as angels, spirit guides, and deceased ancestors. They can also visually perceive the color of someone's aura.

CLAIRCOGNIZANCE: CLEAR KNOWING

Have you ever just known something was true, seemingly out of the blue? Claircognizance is when information you otherwise wouldn't know just seems to pop into your brain! No other senses brought you this information, nothing happened for you to deduce the truth—*you just knew* in a prophetic way. When something swoops into your awareness and seems to nag at you until you acknowledge it, this is considered "clear knowing" and it is a favorite way of the spiritual world to communicate with us.

CLAIRAUDIENCE: CLEAR HEARING

This one can be the most frightening, as our society places a huge stigma on "hearing voices," associating it with psychosis. But clairaudience is simply perceiving sounds, words, phrases, or music from the ethereal world. The voice may sound as if it's inside your head, spoken right nearby but outside of your head, or even echoing, as if from another dimension. If you intermittently experience ringing in your ears—not for a long period of time, but in short spurts, particularly when focusing on spiritual practices— this could be a sign of developing clairaudience and Spirit trying to get through to you.

CLAIRSENTIENCE: CLEAR PHYSICAL FEELING

Many renowned spiritual communicators can *feel* the physical experience of others or spiritual beings in their body. Someone with clairsentience can be with a friend who has an ailment or injury and literally feel their pain in the same location on their own body. The same is true for a deceased person in the spirit world. For example, if a person died from a gunshot to the head, the spiritual medium might exerience a sudden splitting headache while communicating with them.

CLAIRSALIENCE: CLEAR SMELLING

With clairsalience, insights from the spirit world come to you via the perception of smell. If you often smell the cologne of your deceased grandfather yet no one in your home wears anything close to it, that is an example of clear smelling. It also means your grandfather loves hanging around you!

CLAIRTANGENCY: CLEAR TOUCHING

Also commonly known as psychometry, clairtangency is the extrasensory perception that allows someone to know things otherwise unknown to them about certain objects or people by simply touching them. If you've ever just known the history of something you've picked up at a flea market or secondhand shop, that is clear touching and it is quite a gift!

CLAIRGUSTANCE: CLEAR TASTING

The ability to taste things in your mouth when there is nothing there is clairgustance. An example would be tasting your deceased grandmother's spaghetti recipe (yum!) long after she has passed, indicating, of course, that she is near you.

CLAIREMPATHY: CLEAR EMOTIONAL FEELING

If you've been called an empath, you probably possess the power of clairempathy. Sensing other people's emotions, thoughts, and energy defines this extrasensory perception. When you walk into a room after a couple has been arguing and feel the emotions without having seen or heard the argument beforehand, that is clairempathy.

How Spirit Communicates with Us

Medium Susanne Wilson says that "spirit communication is like water. It follows the path of least resistance." That's why children are often the natural receivers of communication from Spirit. It's also why the more we open our hearts and minds to Spirit, the more it will invest in getting personalized messages to us. Below are some of the ways in which our spirit teams like to communicate with us.

MATERIALIZATIONS

Feathers falling to us out of nowhere, coins appearing on the sidewalk with significant dates, electrical anomalies (i.e., flickering lights), meaningful music randomly popping on the radio, a double rainbow on your birthday—these are all ways Spirit, particularly our deceased ancestors, manipulate the dense material energy of our world to bring us messages that let us know they are nearby.

NUMBERS

Have you ever noticed repeating numbers that continually show up in your life, such as 1111, 1234, 888, etc.? Pay attention to them, because often they contain important and specific messages from your angels, guides, and ancestors. See the chapter on numerology about how numbers explain literally everything—when certain patterns or repeating numbers relentlessly show up in your life, it's time to listen! Also, note that while it's easy and fun to Google what certain number patterns mean, it's best to first think of what the numbers mean to you when they keep showing up. Never forget that all the answers are inside you.

SYNCHRONICITIES

You've experienced synchronicity. We all have. When everything lines up just perfectly: the right time, the right place, the right people in front of you. The average person calls this a "coincidence" or "chance," but we don't believe there is such a thing!

When things fall so effortlessly into place in a synchronistic fashion, that is your spirit team telling you that you are on the right path, in sync with the natural laws of the universe, and thus, that they are helping orchestrate magic in your life. Conversely, if you experience setback after setback with zero synchronicities, it's merely the universe's way of redirecting you to what is in alignment with your highest self. It's beneficial to change your mind-set in these moments of seeming rejection from "Why me?" to "What's the lesson here for me?" When you start to pay attention to what's paying attention to you, you'll begin to understand what your spirit team is trying to communicate.

ANIMAL MESSENGERS

While the spirit world often uses the elements to get messages to us, our spirit team also joins in with the animal kingdom. Animals work with the spirit world to protect, teach, and deliver messages to humans. Whether it's a jaguar or a skunk or your favorite rare bird, animals are often sent to us as messengers from our spirit teams who are trying to bring us deeper insights on our life's path. This also includes magical creatures like dragons, mermaids, and fairies!

If you see an animal out of the blue, or some mention or image of a specific animal keeps coming into your life, and in your gut you feel it's something more than just "being in the right place at the right time," then there is probably a message for you from this animal. Before looking up what that animal spirit is said to mean by ancient tribes and modern shamans, meditate on it quietly and see what pops up in your mind. This is an excellent way to learn to trust more in your intuition and spirit team's guidance.

DREAM VISITS

Dream visits from the spirit world are well documented in ancient texts. The Egyptians had a large focus on the dream world, as they considered dreams to be direct messages from the gods. The Bible even mentions how the three wise men were "warned by a dream" to depart on a different road than they originally intended after visiting baby Jesus, to avoid confrontation or danger. And in the book of Genesis, Jacob had a fateful dream in which he saw a staircase going up to heaven, with angels ascending and descending.

Whether by our spirit guides, angels, or ancestors, dream visits are one of the most popular ways in which Spirit chooses to communicate with us. This is because it is in our dream state that our subconscious minds are most susceptible to the alternative realms of existence and the most impressionable to messages from the world of Spirit. How many times have you woken up knowing the solution to a problem you had struggled with just the day before? We can thank our spirit team for those epiphanies.

Before I went to bed one night, I asked my mother, who had recently died of Alzheimer's, to come to me in a dream. I hadn't heard her voice in five years, even though she had just died two months before. That night, in my dream, a door opened and my mother walked into my room. I heard her voice as clear as day. She told me that even when she couldn't speak, she had always been communicating with me. When I woke up, I felt her presence with me.

—*Louise, 48*

Make a Date with Your Spirit Team

Did you know you don't have to wait for your spirit team to visit you in your sleep—you can organize a visit? This prescription for having a dream visit from your guides, angels, or ancestors was written by spiritual medium Susanne Wilson in her book *Soul Smart: What the Dead Teach Us about Spirit Communication.*

• Choose one night per week and ask for a dream visit that night. Let your loved one in spirit know. Extend an invitation to them in your mind by saying something like, *"(Name), on Sunday night I'm inviting you for a dream visit. Please come!"*

• On the night of the appointment, light a candle and meditate. Then place the following items near your bed:

  • A plain glass or bowl of water, because water is a spirit conductor.
  • A picture of your loved one.
  • A personal item that had belonged to your loved one.

• Just before falling asleep, focus on a happy memory with that loved one; avoid thoughts that bring pain or grief.

• Ask for the gift of a dream visit and ask for the gift of remembering the dream. Ask your angels to help as well.

• When you first awaken, close your eyes and allow your mind to drift a little. This is the best time to remember your dream visit. Write down what you remember in a dream journal as soon as you can.

• Last, but not least: give gratitude for the visit, but of course!

PAST LIFE REGRESSION

"As a man, casting off worn-out garments, takes new ones, so the dweller in the body, casting off worn-out bodies, enters into others that are new."

—*Bhagavad Gita*

Have you ever connected so quickly with a new friend that you felt like you'd known each other forever? Or taken an instant dislike to someone you just barely met? Or had a mentor who felt more like a mother or father figure to you? It's possible you knew all these people in a past life.

Family groups tend to reincarnate together over many lifetimes until we learn the lessons from each other that we need to learn. So that friend who feels more like a sister may have been your sister in a previous life. The person you instantly hate could have been someone who once wronged you, while that fatherly professor may have been your parent. The question is: What are you meant to learn from them?

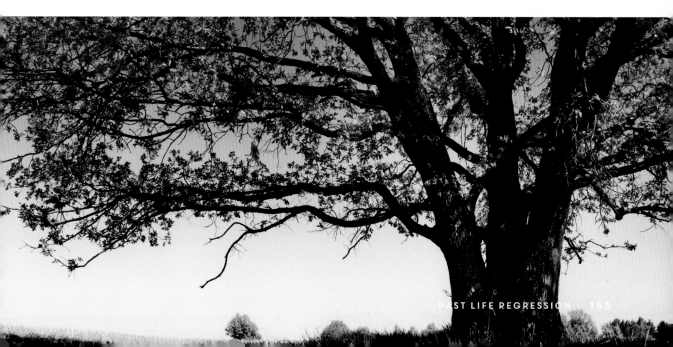

What Is Past Life Regression?

The subject of reincarnation is nothing new. Reincarnation is a tenet in many religions, including Buddhism, Hinduism, Jainism, and Sikhism. Other religions, such as Christianity, Islam, and some pagan belief systems, believe in an afterlife, where the soul continues to exist in another realm after death. The ancient Greeks believed that the soul was reincarnated after death and the body was merely a vessel for the soul in each lifetime.

In order to explore the reincarnations of our soul, we use a healing therapy known as past life regression. The word *regression* means a going back to, or a return to, something. Past life regression, then, means to go back to the far reaches of our subconscious mind, where our soul's history of many lifetimes is recorded. Exploring the soul's past journey brings deeper meaning to our present life and can also reveal insights for our future. By examining our past lives, regression work can help us heal our past traumas in this present lifetime.

Whether we're talking about past incarnations or just this one life we are experiencing now, we know that history repeats itself. There is no doubt that our past—our childhood, our birth, even our time in the womb—can greatly affect us throughout our life. If we don't examine our pasts, our futures will be laced with the same traumas and challenges that we've seen before. But we aren't meant to keep experiencing the same hurtful patterns; we are meant to grow from our past, transcend our limitations, and blossom into the most loving, self-actualized version of ourselves.

"The soul incarnates and experiences often death. The bodies are like glasses for the Soul, which gradually, life after life must be filled. First the mud glass, then the wooden glass, soon after the glass ones and finally the silver and golden glass."

—*Origen of Alexandria*

Scientific Data

Is there really any science behind this? Many proponents of past life regression say yes.

Perhaps the most respected collection of scientific data that strongly points to proof that reincarnation is real is the research of Dr. Ian Stevenson. Devoting most of his life to this research, Dr. Stevenson methodically documented patients' (mostly children's) statements of a previous lifetime. He then identified the deceased person the child remembered being, and verified the facts of the deceased person's life that matched the child's memory—including physical things, such as birthmarks, birth defects, wounds, and scars on the deceased, which were all corroborated by medical records. He was strict in his methods so as to confidently rule out all other possible explanations for the child's past life recollections. The results? With more than 3,000 cases in his files, many people, including skeptics and scholars, agree that Stevenson's research offers the best evidence yet for reincarnation.

A physician who trained at Columbia and Yale, Dr. Brian Weiss has made contributions to the field of past life regression that have earned him the nickname "father of modern past life regression." Weiss is a psychiatrist who did not believe in reincarnation; however, in the process of treating a patient named Catherine using conventional psychotherapy and hypnosis, Dr. Weiss heard Catherine discuss details of a past life. As a skeptic about reincarnation, Dr. Weiss spent much time confirming elements of Catherine's stories through public records, and after seeing the undeniable truth in them, he became convinced of the survival of the human personality after death. Since his first surprise experience with Catherine, Dr. Weiss claims to have conducted successful past life regressions with 4,000 clients since 1980. He continued to use past life regression in Catherine's follow-up treatments and the results were nothing short of miraculous. He published his experiences in detail in his first book, *Many Lives, Many Masters*, which has become the most widely read book about past life regression therapy to date.

"Every time you are tempted to react in the same old way, ask if you want to be a prisoner of the past or a pioneer of the future."

—*Deepak Chopra*

HOW IT WORKS

In the practical sense of past life regression, a trained hypnosis and regression professional guides you to review a past life or lives using hypnosis, creative visualization, meditation, reverie, and other methods. A regression hypnosis period typically lasts about one and a half hours, and multiple lifetimes can be reviewed in one session. It's an interactive process, with the practitioner asking questions and guiding the session to help you uncover your subconscious wisdom.

There are also audio recordings that can guide you through the process as well as other tools you can use yourself, such as automatic writing. However, be aware that some of the information you uncover can be quite painful and is best explored with a trained professional.

So how does it work, exactly? The subconscious communicates with us through imagery, symbols, and metaphors; when we explore these deep aspects of our subconscious through hypnosis or guided visualization, our inner knowing is revealed to us. We may finally understand the unhelpful patterns we keep repeating or why we have certain phobias, negative emotions, or limiting beliefs. We also know that emotional trauma can lodge in the body, become trapped, and cause physical pain; understanding the root causes of that trauma can release the pain. The process can also clear negative karma (the sum of your actions in previous lives) and release you from past life contracts that you no longer need to maintain, removing energy blocks that are keeping you stuck. Finally, by uncovering your subconscious wisdom, past life regression helps you align with your soul's purpose in this lifetime—the lessons you need to learn in order to release their hold on you.

My client, Adriana, came to see me after a trip to Egypt. She had been on a guided tour of an ancient tomb when she had an intense knowing that she had been a slave buried there in a past life. She was so overcome by a feeling of suffocation and constriction in her throat that she had a severe panic attack.

It was clear that her feelings of enslavement from a past life had followed her into this one. She felt restricted by her parents and her tendency to follow their rules of life rather than her own. As we worked together, she began to take risks that others might not approve of, such as pursuing her creative side, and started to find some "breathing room" in her constricted relationships and work life. You could say that the shackles from her past life as a slave in Egypt were thrown off in this one and she was finally free to shine as the person she was always meant to be.

—*Ellen*, past life regression therapist

Can we verify that Adriana was actually a slave buried in a tomb in Egypt long ago? No. But did the process of past life regression help her? Absolutely. She came to understand the repeating patterns in her life, the source of her emotional pain, and why she felt stuck. She was able to view her childhood experiences in a new light and to understand why she reacted to her parents the way she did.

Adriana's feelings of enslavement and suffocation may have been metaphors from her subconscious, trying to get her to pay attention to her innermost feelings. Regardless of whether these metaphors were linked to an actual historical fact, they had a resonant emotional truth for her and opened a path to self-discovery and growth.

Astrology and Past Lives

If you recall the discussion of the north and south nodes in the astrology chapter, the south node position indicates the skills, talents, and psychological patterns and habits you developed in previous incarnations. These, in turn, are the traits in which you feel most comfortable and confident in your current lifetime. The south node placement is your ultimate comfort zone. Many astrologers say that the south node also indicates where we might have got things wrong in our past lives and can warn us how to avoid self-destruction in this current lifetime. If you're interested in learning about your past lives, studying your south node placement is a good place to start.

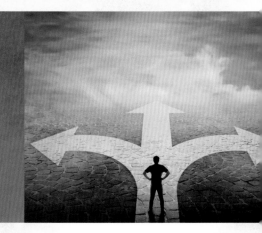

"Only we can rid ourselves ... of the bad habits that we accumulate when we are in a physical state. The Masters cannot do that for us. If you choose to fight and not to rid yourself, then you will carry them over into another life. And only when you decide that you are strong enough to master the external problems, then you will no longer have them in your next life."

—*Dr. Brian Weiss*, Many Lives, Many Masters

"For one who has taken birth, death is certain and for one who has died, birth is certain."

—*Bhagavad Gita*

> "We can predict the future, when we know how the present moment evolved from the past."
>
> —*Carl Jung*

Life Between Lives

There has recently been a new development in regression therapy called Life Between Lives (LBL) regression. LBL is described as a deep hypnotic process that reconnects you with your soul self and your guiding beings, such as guardian angels. This leads to an understanding of your immortal identity, the personality that is reborn again and again.

Like past life regression, LBL is experienced through a profound hypnotic regression. However, instead of examining past incarnations, you journey to the time your soul spends in the spirit world *between* incarnations. During LBL regression, you'll experience yourself as an immortal soul, meet your guides and deceased loved ones, and review your soul lessons and life purpose for this lifetime.

No matter which method you use, past life regression is an ultimately empowering process. It leads to greater self-understanding and deep healing in a way that no other therapy can accomplish so quickly. By examining the past, it allows you to take control of your life in the here and now.

Signs of a Past Life

Is your soul trying to tell you something? Is there a past life you need to explore? Here are some ways to know:

- You have vivid, repeating dreams about a person you don't know or a place you've never been

- You have a natural talent for something that no one in your family has

- You keep repeating the same painful pattern in relationships

- You are drawn to collect specific objects and don't know why

- You are irrationally afraid of a specific way of dying or of someone you love dying that way

- You are magnetically drawn to, or repelled by, someone you just met

- You are drawn to a particular place or time in history

- You have a strong connection to, or an irrational fear of, a specific animal

- You are obsessed with someone or something that you can't explain

- You have experienced déjà vu

- You know how to speak a language you've never been exposed to

- You are triggered by a sound or smell that has no basis in your current life

- You have knowledge about a subject you have never studied

MEDIUMSHIP

"Death is not real, even in the relative sense–it is but birth to a new life–and you shall go on, and on, and on, to higher and still higher planes of life."

—*The Kybalion*

There is a truth about dying, and it's a truth that, when understood, is the greatest informant in living our absolute best lives. Everyone wants to live a free, abundant, creative, and authentic life, yet there is much misery in the world because our society is not set up for freedom, abundance, creativity, and authenticity. Instead, society revolves around all kinds of fear-based thinking, the fear of death being the big one. And fear debilitates us.

The truth about dying is this: *we don't die.* And understanding this truth is the ultimate one-way ticket to freedom in life.

Ask yourself: *How would you live if you knew you did not really die?* As afterlife researchers, we can assure you that the eternal nature of our soul is indeed the truth. The ancient mystics, priests, priestesses, and sages unanimously believed that death is but the beginning of a new life. Thanks to popular TV shows like *Crossing Over with John Edwards* and *Long Island Medium*, most people today have at least a superficial idea of what mediumship is. It's the ability to communicate, in one way or another, with those who have passed over. A "medium" is literally the midpoint between a deceased spirit and a living person, communicating messages from the former to the latter.

Mediumship is an important healing tool because, more than anything, it convinces us what our ancestors have always known: life is eternal. And when we understand the truth in that, we can then begin living our lives the way they were meant to be lived: fearlessly and authentically.

Mediumship Across Time and Space

Although it didn't become popular until the 19th century with the Spiritualist movement, mediumship has deep, ancient roots. Necromancy, Greek for "divination of the dead," is the magical practice of summoning spirits to gain knowledge about the future. In ancient societies, it was thought that the spirits of the deceased had vital knowledge that could be communicated to the living through specific rituals.

Probably the society best known for communing with, and honoring, the dead was ancient Egypt. The ancient Egyptians considered a person's life on Earth to be only one part of an eternal journey—believing that while the personality was created at the time of physical birth, the soul was an immortal entity inhabiting a mortal vessel for a short ride. When that vessel died physically, the ancient Egyptians believed that the soul transformed to another plane of existence, the afterlife.

Native Americans are well known for having a strong reverence for ancestors, and many medicine men are mystics who possess the ability to leave their body and communicate with the spirit world.

And though Christianity overarchingly denounces mediumship now, it was not immune to mediumship in the ancient era. In fact, some say the entire religion was indeed built on a foundation of mediumship! For what else was Jesus but a highly advanced medium? He is accepted to have been a master communicator with Spirit and a profound healer. He also taught that death was the beginning of eternal life.

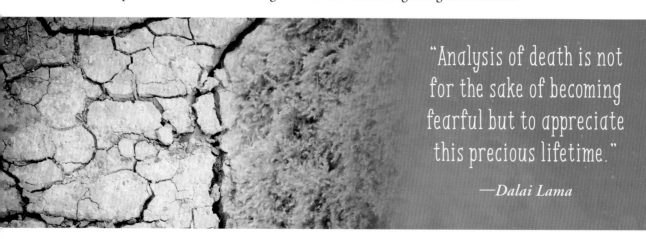

"Analysis of death is not for the sake of becoming fearful but to appreciate this precious lifetime."

—*Dalai Lama*

What *Is* a Medium?

Every serious religion has had a serious interest in the afterlife, and thus every culture from prehistoric to modern times has had men and women who claimed to have the gift of mediumship. Medicine men, shamans, oracles, and witches were all called upon to maintain contact with the spirit world for the whole of the clan, tribe, or society.

So, what *is* a medium, exactly? A medium is a person with heightened extrasensory perceptions that allow them to be, literally, a medium between the ethereal spirit world and our physical world. People in Spirit vibrate at a much higher frequency than we living folks do. In order to bridge the gap and make a connection, a spiritual medium needs to raise his or her own vibration higher, and Spirit has to lower its vibration as well so the two can meet in the middle, allowing the medium to be a mouthpiece for the deceased. Via clairvoyance (clear seeing), clairaudience (clear hearing), claircognizance (clear knowing), clairsentience (clear feeling), and other methods, mediums are able to download information from the deceased and then relay, first, the evidence that it is truly they, and then, whatever message the spirit has for the living person receiving the reading.

There are various kinds of mediumships, with mental mediumship, physical mediumship, and trance mediumship being the three giants. Mental mediumship communicates with the spirit world through telepathy. Physical mediumship manipulates energy and energy systems of spirits, and it is manifested in the physical world, such as by sudden loud noises, disembodied voices, and material objects doing immaterial things, such as levitating. Trance mediumship is when the medium goes into a trance and Spirit uses the person's voice to communicate messages.

Although each type of mediumship communicates with Spirit in unique ways, the important point is that a medium delivers messages from the deceased. Often, these messages aid in healing deep grief and allow the grieving person to feel a continuing connection with the deceased. To know that our loved one lives on can bring the deepest healing and peace.

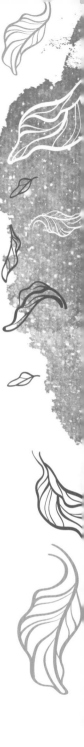

How to Sit for a Mediumship Reading

When it comes to mediumship readings, there are things you should and should not do to make your reading successful.

DO:

1. **Get relaxed.** It's totally normal to be nervous before a reading with a medium. Before you go, either meditate or do whatever helps you slip into a state of chill.

2. **Write out your questions before your appointment.** This is simply so you don't stress out trying to "remember" what you wanted to say to your deceased loved ones; this will reduce anxiety and help you maintain a relaxed state.

3. **Record the session.** Amnesia after your reading is a real thing, and you'll want to record everything your loved one in the spirit world has to say! Playing the recording back, even years later, can still evoke the same feelings and potential for healing.

DON'T:

1. **Drink alcohol.** Drinking alcohol, being hung over, or using drugs or other intoxicating substances the day of your reading is a no-no. These things all lower our vibrations and a reading demands everyone's highest vibes!

2. **Feed the medium.** While you should use your voice to say yes and no (because our loved ones in Spirit love hearing our voices!), if the medium asks whether you recognize or acknowledge any of the messages coming through, you should not give information about your life. If a medium asks a lot of questions, this is called fishing and it's a red flag. You should not be giving them more information than they give you!

3. **Force messages that don't fit.** If something the medium says doesn't make total sense, tell him or her that. No good comes from trying to make a message fit when it doesn't—not for the medium, not for you, and not for Spirit.

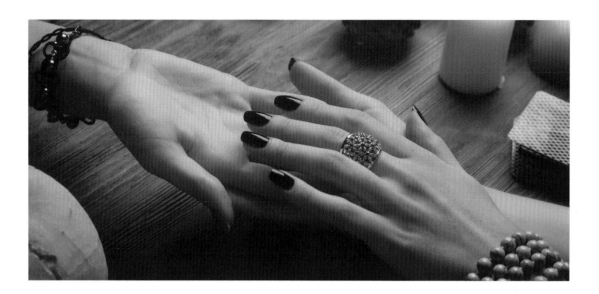

How Mediumship Messages Come Through

When a medium contacts Spirit, it generally happens in three phases. In the first phase, Spirit is entering the medium's energy field and drawing closer to his or her consciousness. The messages the medium receives at this stage will likely have little meaning for them, but as they begin to communicate the message to the sitter, Spirit learns that the medium is able to communicate what Spirit wishes to communicate.

The next phase begins as Spirit and medium maintain a strong connection and Spirit transmits a clearer message to the medium. This part tends to be more easily understood and may be delivered quickly and succinctly.

When Spirit is satisfied that the message has been understood, it begins to withdraw, initiating the third phase. The message becomes a little less clear as the link with Spirit becomes weaker. Finally, the message ends as the energy fields separate.

"Birth is not the beginning of life—only of an individual awareness. Change into another state is not death—only the ending of this awareness."

—Hermes Trismegistus

Cultivating Your Mediumship Abilities

All of us are born with psychic abilities. Think about the times you "knew" something without any physical information: maybe you knew who was calling before you picked up the phone, or you sensed when something terrible had happened to a loved one.

While some people shrug off this psychic ability as "coincidence," other people are drawn to it and develop their psychic intuition. In order to tune in to your "soul frequency," the quiet voice of your intuition, you first need to turn down the noise of the outside world. You can do this through meditation, journaling, maintaining periods of silence, taking a mindful walk in nature, or some other process that works for you. Once you have strengthened your psychic abilities, you are ready to try connecting with Spirit.

Spirit communication often takes place in images and symbols, and it is up to the medium to be able to translate this in a meaningful way for the sitter. Again, this is where intuition comes in; the symbol or image might not mean anything to you, but if you align your inner knowing with the message coming through, you can translate it in a way that is meaningful for the sitter.

Remember that the medium needs to vibrate at a higher frequency in order to meet the spirit world, which will need to lower its vibration. It's hard at first to be able to maintain this high vibration for long enough to make contact. It is not unusual to become too exhausted or unable to focus long enough to maintain this high frequency. This is where practice, patience, and hard work come in. Here are some ways to develop your mediumship:

- Study with a reputable medium in a group of like-minded people. This is known as a "development" or "spirit" circle. The medium knows how to assist the unfoldment process. The circle should work with one kind of mediumship so that all the group's energy is directed in the same way.
- Follow a guided meditation, either an audiotape for this purpose or in a spirit circle, to relax your mind and open your awareness of, and sensitivity to, Spirit. This takes time and patience, and it's good to mix up the exercises so that you challenge yourself to go beyond your limitations.

- Create a weekly time and place to make your appointment with Spirit.
- Do not eat food or drink caffeine before your appointed time, because they can ground you too much in the body or act as a stimulant.
- If you are in a spirit circle, do not discuss your spirit messages with others. This can bring a level of analytical thinking into what is a transcendent experience and can muddy the waters the next time you are seeking to get a message from Spirit.
- Cultivate a course of study of mediumship in addition to your channeling work, either in a group, online, in a course, or by reading reputable material.
- Make sure to learn the ethics of mediumship readings, as you are delivering sensitive information to often grieving people, and integrity is the most important part of the job.

Let the Golden Rule, Rule You

When life gets stressful and difficult, many of us come to wonder what the point of this human existence is anyway. Mediumship throughout the ages has unanimously informed us about some chief purposes of human existence. To treat others as you would like to be treated—aka the Golden Rule—is the number one takeaway of all true mediums across all of time. Kindness, compassion, and forgiveness are the keys to all the locks.

The incentive for practicing the "be kind" mantra goes beyond just niceties—it is, in fact, for our own self-interest: all of the most profound mediums tell us that our vibration in this life dictates our vibration in the next one, and the best way to increase our vibes is through love, kindness, compassion, and forgiveness. We get the afterlife experience we deserve based on how we live our life in the here and now.

TAROT

"The tarot is an outer oracle of which the inner oracle is the source."

—*Philippe St. Genoux*

Imagine that all you need to know is already inside you. Tarot is the magical key that can unlock this wisdom to guide you on your journey through life! A deck of tarot cards is a powerful divination tool. This little collection of cards can help you bypass the intellect of verbal language and thinking processes and directly access your intuition and inner wisdom.

There are many versions of tarot decks in various artistic styles, but they all contain symbols and archetypes that are recognized by the subconscious mind. That's because the cards contain a collective, universal wisdom that aligns with your Higher Self and your inner knowing. Because tarot depicts universal themes and emotions, every spiritual lesson you meet in your life is represented in the deck. Consulting tarot cards helps you see which lesson you might need to learn at a particular moment in time, allowing you to tap into your inner wisdom, bring that wisdom into your conscious awareness, and manifest your goals. It is an empowering practice that lets you access Spirit and your Higher Self as a source of insight and compassion.

Make no mistake: tarot does not "foretell" your future and a tarot practitioner does not "explain" your cards. A practitioner simply guides you to look at the cards and describe what images or feelings are revealed in them. Using insightful queries and a knowledge of the cards' symbolism, the practitioner helps you explore the themes and insights that emerge from the cards. If you'd rather be your own guide, and you are willing to put the work in, you don't need a practioner at all. There are many books, websites, classes, and other guides that can help you understand each card's symbolism and how they work together, an education that can set you free for a lifetime of practice.

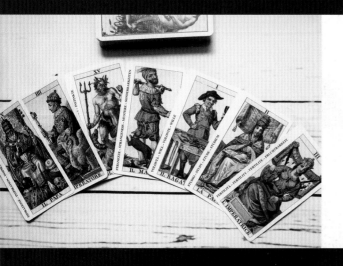

"The tarot represents the spectrum of the human condition, the good, the evil, the light, and the dark. Do not fear the darker aspects of the human condition. Understand them."

—*Benebell Wen*, HOLISTIC TAROT

When I pulled the 'Mother of Wands' card, the image of the coiled snake wrapped around eggs spoke to me in my role as a mother protecting my children. That was all well and good when my children were babies and needed safeguarding, but now I had teenagers chafing at my overprotectiveness. I realized that too much constriction in that snake's tense coil could break the fragile eggs within. It was then that I realized I needed to release my grasp on my teenagers yearning for freedom and growth. I had to relax my coil around them or I would shatter their burgeoning confidence, and our relationship. The 'wand' in the image means to me that I am the orchestrator of my own life, not a passive recipient.

—*Jessica*, age 49

Major Arcana and Minor Arcana

———— • ————

In practical terms, a tarot deck contains 78 cards, and each card
has its own number, imagery, and symbolism. The deck has two
subsets: 22 Major Arcana cards and 56 Minor Arcana cards,
which represent "greater secrets" and "lesser secrets."

MAJOR ARCANA CARDS

The Major Arcana are rich with symbolism and are connected to many spiritual keys,
including:

- A pathway on the Tree of Life in Qabalah
- Chakras on the 12-chakra system
- Gemstones and crystals
- Astrological signs and planets
- Sacred geometry
- Angels and spirit guides
- Egyptian and Hermetic mythology
- Numerology

There are many ways to interpret the Major Arcana cards, but many people associate
them with larger life questions, archetypes, and spiritual quests. These cards are more
dominant in a reading and depict the journey of the psyche, starting with "the Fool"
(numbered 0) and ending with "the World" (numbered XXI). If you think about it, we
are all "fools" at birth, with no knowledge or sense. Hopefully at the end of our lifetime,
we have become one with the world, part of the larger cosmos and at peace with our
place in it.

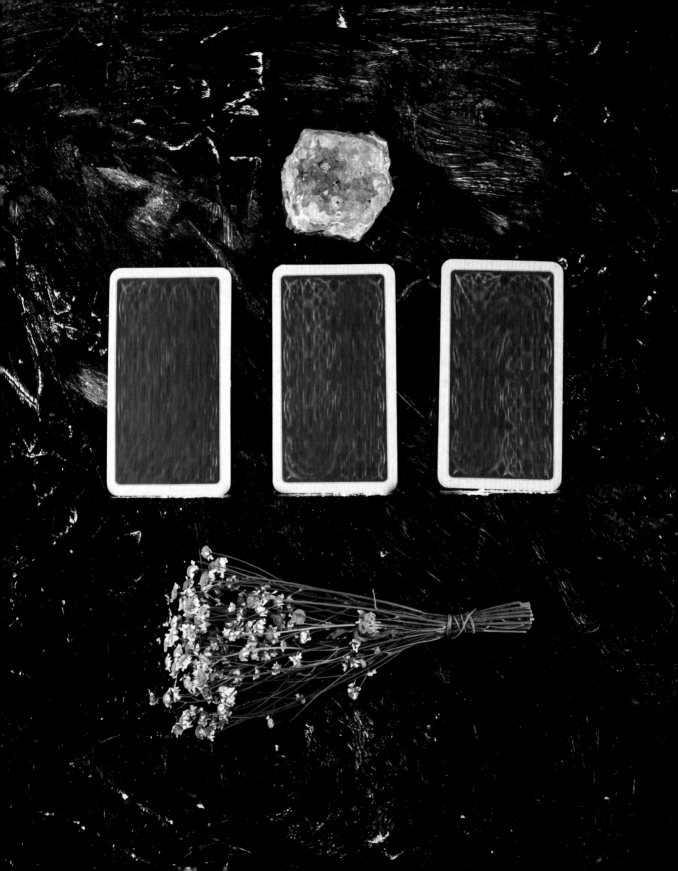

The Major Arcana are spiritual signposts marking the major transitions in life:

0 THE FOOL: The beginning and the end. A free spirit that lives in innocence and spontaneity.

1 THE MAGICIAN: "As above, so below" is the mantra of the Magician. The Magician is pure potential, creativity, resourcefulness, and has a concentration on the path ahead.

2 THE HIGH PRIESTESS: Balance, forethought before action, and intuition. The High Priestess is also known for her connection to the subconscious mind and the Divine Feminine.

3 THE EMPRESS: Nurturing and maternity are embodied in The Empress, as well as femininity, nature, abundance, and success in family matters.

4 THE EMPEROR: Masculinity, structure, and authority are represented in The Emperor. He is the Father Figure of the Major Arcana and embodies stability.

5 THE HIEROPHANT: Akin to the Pope or spiritual leader, The Hierophant is the complementary card to The High Priestess and is sometimes named as such. He represents conformity, learning, and the importance of spirituality/religion in life.

6 THE LOVERS: Love, relationships, harmony, duality, and understanding are represented in this beautiful card.

7 THE CHARIOT: Willpower, success, determination, and forward motion are the gifts of The Chariot. Also, strength in the face of challenges.

8 JUSTICE: Law, integrity, fairness, truth, and decision-making. The Justice card represents cause and effect. Can also be number 11 in some decks.

9 THE HERMIT: Solitude, soul-searching, reflection, introspection, inner guidance, mysticism, and realization are represented in The Hermit card. Go within to find.

10 WHEEL OF FORTUNE: Luck, fate, destiny, turning point, and karma are represented in The Wheel of Fortune. Quite literally, a fortunate opportunity or scenario.

11 STRENGTH: Fortitude, courage, control, discipline, self-mastery, and resilience. The Strength can also be number 8 in some decks.

12 THE HANGED MAN: Crossroads, surrender, new perspective, change, letting go, sacrifice. Change is good and this card allows for a pause to see a new way.

13 DEATH: The most feared and misunderstood card in the deck, The Death card signifies new beginnings. For one thing to begin, another must die. Change and transformation. It's not a death sentence!

14 TEMPERANCE: Moderation, self-control, balance, purpose, patience. A welcomed stop on the path to enlightenment after The Death card. A slow and deliberate new beginning.

15 THE DEVIL: The shadow self, materialism, ignorance, addiction, attachment. This card is a reminder of the evils and temptations of straying from our connection to Spirit.

16 THE TOWER: Sudden change that jolts you out of a pattern or situation. Feared but necessary, this change comes as chaos, an awakening, and a revelation. Not always easy, but vital.

17 THE STAR: Calmess (after the storm of The Tower), spirituality, brilliance, hope, faith, inspiration, and a renewal of purpose.

18 THE MOON: Lack of clarity, illusion, fear, uncertainty, the beginning of understanding, sensitivities, dreams, psychic powers. The Moon addresses the deep realms of the subconscious.

19 THE SUN: Blessings, positivity, warmth, playfulness, optimism, joy, vibration, elevation. The Sun is the source of life, and this card is all about abundance.

20 JUDGMENT: Judgment, rebirth, awakening, absolution, a release of negative thoughts, the outcome of choice.

21 THE WORLD: Fulfillment, accomplishment, integration, travel, and the culmination (to begin again) of the "journey of the fool."

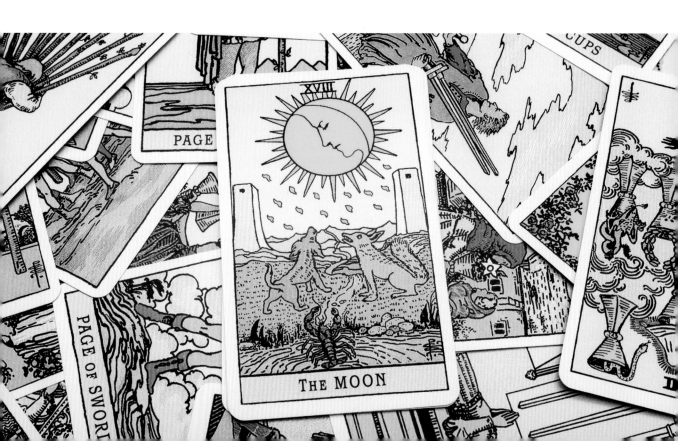

MINOR ARCANA CARDS

The Minor Arcana cards are often assoicated with situations you experience in your everyday life. The Minor Arcana cards can clarify the daily context in which your spiritual quests (Major Arcana) play out. The Minor Arcana contain four suits with 14 cards in each. Cards numbered 1 through 10 depict a situation or an issue you are facing, while the remaining four cards in the suit (known as the "Court cards") often represent people in your life, whether in the past, present, or future.

Court cards can also represent personality traits or tendencies within you, rather than real people. The Court cards are often depicted as the Page, Knight, Queen, and King, but are not to be mistaken for, or associated with, gender. These royal ranks can also be considered a stage of life, rather than a person: the Page is early childhood, the Knight is adolescence, the Queen is the yin (or "feminine") side of adulthood, and the King is the yang (or "masculine") side of adulthood. These cards are often difficult to grasp and require a lot of intuition and symbolism to understand their meaning, but as you work with them, they will become clearer in the context of your own readings.

THE CARDS OF THE MINOR ARCANA ARE:

1/ACE: New beginning, pure potential, great opportunity, birth

2: Duality, balance, attraction, partnership

3: Growth, creativity, cooperation, fruitfulness, expansion

4: Stability, security, manifestation, strong foundation

5: Challenge, change, instability, fluctuations, issues, loss

6: Harmony, peace, cooperation, comfort, healing, regaining stability

7: Assessment, spirituality, reflection, discovery, accomplishment

8: Progress, self-mastery, motivation, accomplishment, fortitude

9: Awakening, fruition, achievement, attainment, self-knowledge

10: Renewal, endings, beginnings, the pause between states

PAGE: The Page is the youngest in the court cards and can represent newness and a fresh perspective, or literally children in your life.

KNIGHT: Represented by younger men in traditional decks, the Knight acts decisively and rashly.

QUEEN: The Queen is the matriarch and caregiver. She represents protection, love, and care.

KING: As the leader of the monarchy, the King represents authority and control.

The Four Suits

—————— • ——————

The four suits in the Minor Arcana cards are the Wands, Cups, Swords, and Pentacles. The following chart shows the element associated with each suit, as well as what the suit represents.

SUIT	ELEMENT	ASTROLOGICAL CORRESPONDENCE	REPRESENTS
Wands	Fire	Aries, Leo, and Sagittarius	Spiritual: creativity, the mind
Cups	Water	Cancer, Scorpio, and Pisces	Emotional: relationships
Swords	Air	Gemini, Libra, and Aquarius	Mental: action, conflict, the intellect
Pentacles	Earth	Taurus, Virgo, and Capricorn	Physical: material goods, home, money, career

Each suit can pinpoint the area of your life in which you have questions or are struggling, and it also elucidates the form that inquiry may take. For instance, if you pull a Cups card, you might discern that your emotions are getting the better of you, or that your situation might need to be to be felt with the heart rather than the intellect. If you pull a card with the Swords on it, you might discern that you need to take action to resolve a concern, or maybe that you rely too much on your intellect to guide your way.

When I was fifteen, I was in the midst of adolescent chaos. I was insecure, anxious, and often angry for no reason. Like most teenagers, I slammed doors and stomped around and picked arguments with my parents. At times I felt out of control. A friend who was well versed in tarot gave me a tapestry of the Strength card, and I hung it on my wall. Looking at the girl patting the lion made me feel calm and centered. It wasn't until years later that I learned that the Strength card represents mastering raw emotions in order to bring calm to yourself, which was exactly what I needed to learn at that time.

—*Julia, 23*

How to Do a Tarot Reading

There is no "right way" to do a tarot reading; each person develops their own style and method. There are many tarot decks available, and they each contain their own symbolism and system. It is best to choose a deck that has a style and artistry that resonates with you. Many newbies start with the classic Rider-Waite deck, which is one of the most popular decks and therefore has a lot of background information for the user. The following are some of the most common ways to do a reading.

ASK A QUESTION

Before beginning a reading, it's important to clarify your intention, or what you want to glean from the reading. We have many facets of our lives and threads of people, places, and things woven into the tapestry of our lives. We can't possibly address them all in one (or even several!) readings. It's best to ask a question of the cards so that you can focus your attention and interpretation. Avoid asking yes or no questions. As stated earlier, tarot is not a fortune-telling parlor trick. The purpose of tarot is self-discovery, so focus your question with "what" or "how," such as "What do I need to know about …" or "How can I …"

SHUFFLE THE CARDS

Once you've formulated your question, say it silently or aloud as you shuffle the cards. Shuffling and handling the cards is an important part of the process, because you transfer your energy into the cards and they return awareness and clarity to you. Hold the cards facedown in your nondominant hand (this is considered your "receptive" hand, and you want to be receptive to what the cards can show you). Use your dominant (or "active") hand to pick up cards from the bottom of the deck and place them on top, repeating your question out loud or silently. When you sense you are finished shuffling, stop. It's amazing how people know intuitively when it is time to stop shuffling.

CUT THE CARDS

Place the cards down in front of you. Using your nondominant hand, lift the deck and allow the cards to separate into three piles. Do this intuitively, rather than trying to manipulate the stacks. Then, intuitively combine the three stacks again into one pile.

Different Formats of Readings

There are as many ways to do tarot readings as there are tarot readers, but there are a few common formats that most practitioners use. Which one you'll use on any given day depends on the amount of time you have, how much you want to delve into the cards, and how often you do readings. Once you are comfortable with one format, try the others. One is not better than the others; you can glean just as much understanding from a single-card reading as you can from a full spread.

SINGLE-CARD READING

This is a great way to learn more about the cards and to focus your intention for the day. As you shuffle the cards, ask your question, or if you don't have a burning question, simply ask yourself, "What do I need to know today?" or "What do I need to focus on in my life?" Then either pick the top card from the deck or select one at random. Spend some time looking at the card, reflecting on your question, and discerning the symbolism you find within.

Once you determine how it speaks to you, you can look at the traditional meaning of the card and determine the synthesized message for you. Place the card of the day on your altar, at your desk, on your bathroom mirror, or anywhere that you'll see it throughout the day to remind you of the wisdom, energy, and support of the day's card. If further insight is needed, pull another tarot card to expand the message.

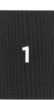

PAST-PRESENT-FUTURE
THREE-CARD SPREAD

This is a sinple spread that is great for beginners and for those who want to understand how a situation might get resolved. Select three cards and lay them facedown. Turn them each over.

CARD 1 = influences from the past that are still affecting you
CARD 2 = the present moment and all that surrounds you
CARD 3 = the future or a likely outcome of your situation

Other ways of reading the cards include, from left to right:

CARD 1 = who I was
CARD 2 = who I am
CARD 3 = who I will be

CARD 1 = context
CARD 2 = focus
CARD 3 = outcome

CARD 1 = what I need to be aware of
CARD 2 = what I need to know now
CARD 3 = what I need to let go of

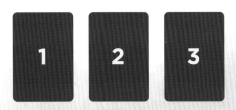

FOUR-CARD CLARITY SPREAD

The four-card clarity spread helps you gain clarity over a situation or an issue. Select four cards and place one at the top and the remaining three in a line below that card.

CARD 1 = the overall situation or issue

CARDS 2, 3, AND 4 = contributing factors to the situation, in no particular order

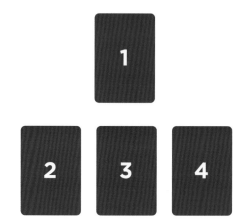

FIVE-CARD CONNECTION SPREAD

This spread is helpful when discerning the dynamics within a relationship and how to meet a challenging situation.

CARD 1 = you

CARD 2 = your challenge

CARD 3 = the other person

CARD 4 = the other person's challenge

CARD 5 = your uniting force

Cards 2 and 4 are the distractions or habits that pull you and the other person apart, respectively; you need to reflect on them. Card 5 holds the key to resolving your challenging situation. It could be your shared vision for the future or your special connection.

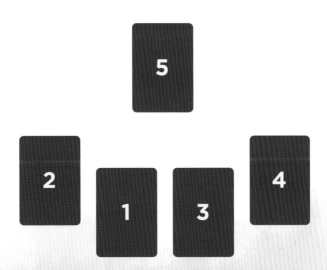

TEN-CARD CELTIC CROSS SPREAD

This is another popular spread. It's complex and delves into all aspects of your situation or issue. It can therefore be a bit overwhelming and is not a spread you should start with. It takes some experience to decipher and can be looked at over a period of days or weeks. Come back to it with fresh eyes and you will see new things each time.

CARD 1 = present situation
CARD 2 = obstacles
CARD 3 = best possible outcome
CARD 4 = root cause
CARD 5 = past
CARD 6 = future
CARD 7 = you right now
CARD 8 = external factors, e.g., family, friends, environment
CARD 9 = hopes and fears
CARD 10 = final outcome

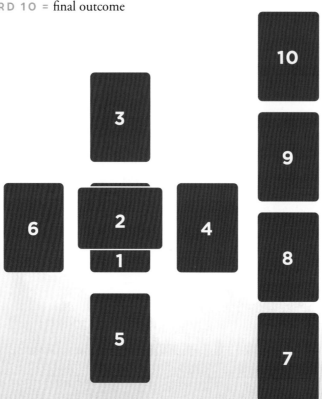

THIRTEEN-CARD YEAR-AHEAD SPREAD

This is an interesting way to explore the year ahead, either on New Year's Eve or on your birthday. Take a photo of the spread so that you can look at it as the year progresses. It is arranged like a clockface with the last card in the center. Each card represents a month, with card 1 being January or your birthday month, however you are doing it. Card 13 represents the overall theme of the year. You can shuffle the deck before you pull each card or pull them all at once, or some other way of your choosing. The spread is not a "prediction" of how your year is going to play out; think of the cards as reminders of what to focus on in the coming months.

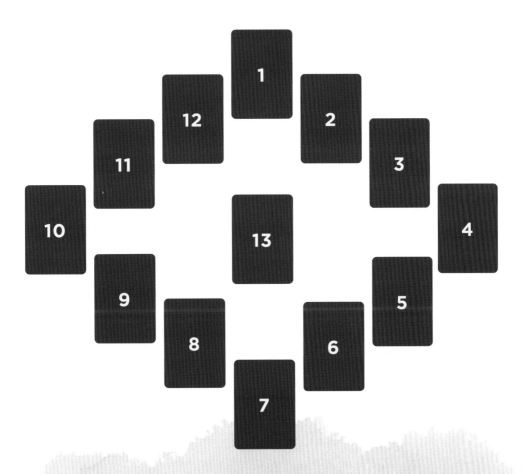

Cleansing Your Cards

Tarot cards pick up the energy of the person handling them. It's important to treat your cards with respect and to keep them in a special place. Handle them with reverence when your mind is open and receptive. Don't use them when you are angry or carrying negative feelings. You'll know when it's time to cleanse your cards—the energy will feel off, you'll be feeling doubt about them, or they'll feel heavy. You also will want to cleanse your cards after lending them to someone, a reading has been very draining, your readings are feeling stagnant or unclear, you haven't used your cards in a long time, or any time you simply wish to reconnect with yor cards.

Here are some ways to cleanse your cards. Use the techniques that feel right for you or your situation:

- **SORTING AND SHUFFLING.** Sort your cards by Major Arcana, then each of the suits of the Minor Arcana. Make sure you aren't missing any cards. Then shuffle them a set number of times (some people choose seven) and infuse them with your positive energy.
- **MEDITATION.** Meditate with your cards. Hold them in your hands, close your eyes, and imagine a universal white light surrounding them.
- **MOON BATH.** Place your cards outside or on a windowsill where they will receive the light of a full moon.
- **SALT BURIAL.** Place your cards in an airtight, zip-top bag and seal it. In an airtight container, place a layer of salt. Place the cards on the salt and then add salt around the sides and over the top, completely covering the cards. Seal the container and leave for a few days. The salt will draw out the impurities.
- **SMUDGE STICK.** Burn some sage or rosemary (or use a smudge stick bought at a store) and pass the cards through the smoke several times.
- **CRYSTAL.** Place a quartz crystal (this crystal absorbs negative energy; see page 28) on top of your cards and place them on a simple altar you make with a cloth, some candles, or other objects that are meaningful to you.

The purpose of the cards is to reveal to you what is already inside you. No one can do that for you. The universal symbology of the cards reminds us that we all face similar obstacles and challenges on our journey. In that sense, no problem or situation is really "new," and you are not as alone or as different as you might think. The more you explore with your cards, the more you will understand about yourself and the direction you want your life to take.

Oracle Cards

Oracle cards are the lawless cousins of tarot and can pretty much be whatever a person wants. Modern oracle cards come in the themes of animals, chakras, crystals, fairies, gods, goddesses, plants, affirmations—almost anything you could think of. Oracle cards are thought to be more for breaking patterns and inspiring intentional change. We like to pull an oracle card to expand upon the meaning of a tarot reading and gain more insight.

SHADOW WORK

"A human being is only breath and shadow."

—Sophocles

Have you ever stumbled upon the tip of an iceberg in your emotional life? Something sparks a strong reaction in you, and you know there's more below the surface, but you tell yourself, "Don't go there." Or perhaps you despise a trait in another person because you can't admit that you harbor similar characteristics. Or maybe in a fit of rage you said something shocking and later thought, "Where did that come from?" Well, it came from you—or more accurately, it came from your shadow side.

The renowned psychiatrist Carl Jung coined the term *shadow* in relation to the human psyche; however, the concept of the shadow self is something ancient cultures knew well—particularly in shamanism, where the shadow is thought of as our greatest teacher.

In ancient Egypt, the soul was thought to consist of several parts, one of which was the shadow of the soul. It makes sense that the Egyptians would recognize the shadow as an important element, considering that they revered the light of the sun and understood the relationship of the shadows it cast. This idea of the same elements of nature reflected in humanity is the essence of the ancient teaching from Hermes "as above, so below" (see the chapter on manifestation, page 56). Just as the dark canvas of the sky is what makes the stars and planets appear so bright, so, too, does the darkness in our own personal lives set the stage for us to shine bright. As writer Thomas Lloyd Qualls said, "Believing you are good is like believing in half the moon." The dark side of the moon isn't visible to us, but that doesn't mean it isn't there.

Just as the sun cannot destroy its shadow, neither can we destroy the shadow within our own souls—and that is not at all the point. We are not meant to battle or attack our dark sides to get rid of them. The goal is to embrace and fully accept our shadows. The shadow does not inherently mean negative or evil, it simply means not yet illuminated.

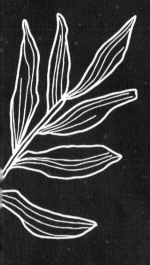

"Everyone carries a shadow, and the less it is embodied in the individual's conscious life, the blacker and denser it is."

—*Carl Jung*

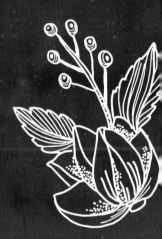

What Is the "Shadow Self"?

———— • ————

Every single day, every single one of us wears a social mask. We put our best, most elevated foot forward in public settings, despite the darker emotions we may be feeling and experiencing internally or in private with our closest loved ones. Of course we do! It's natural to want to look our best and to keep up appearances in an appearance-obsessed, social media–driven world. But beneath that constant "happy" mask, we all have a hidden, wounded, isolated side of our psyche that is called "the shadow," and it represents everything we deny about ourselves.

There is a terrible cost to repressing our shadow self, because eventually the shadow—which so desperately wants to be seen, acknowledged, and soothed—figures out how to pick the lock on its prison cage. And with newfound freedom, it most often chooses to express itself in frightening, explosive, and toxic ways. Whatever is inside of us *will come out*—one way or another. Repressing our darker sides is akin to shaking up a soda bottle over and over. It will inevitably explode when someone finally opens it, and someone *always* opens it.

This is where shadow work comes in. **The shadow is the source of our deepest emotional richness and vitality on our spiritual path. It is meant to be transmuted and harnessed, not avoided.** The more we unapologetically look at and own the shadow sides of ourselves, the more we accept and love ourselves unconditionally, and thus, the more wholehearted and authentic we become.

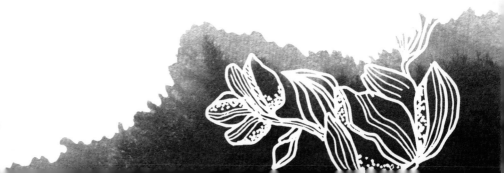

Dark and Golden Shadows

The shadow self is not only the darker elements of
our personalities, such as jealousy, anger, vulnerability,
self-hatred, guilt, and shame, but also the positive
aspects we suppress, such as creativity, personal power,
passion, and spiritual yearnings. These are referred
to, respectively, as dark shadow and golden shadow.
The golden shadow is literally the repressed "gold"
inside of us. It is our unfulfilled potential that we
failed to develop due to the stifling combination
of low self-worth and fear of risk-taking, which
are all tangled up in the dark shadow; therefore,
our golden aspects cannot emerge and bloom in
the light until we first face the dark shadow.

What Is Shadow Work?

Now that we understand what the shadow *is*, the next question is *how* do we bring our repressed shadows to our conscious life? We do it through a healing modality known as *shadow work*. Today, many spiritual healers call themselves "light workers." But we must first be "shadow workers." Why? Because until we do our own personal shadow work, our light work will not be authentic. And no one likes artificial lighting.

When we were children, repressing our darker selves was a method of self-protection—a survival mechanism. We created a shadow side to hold sacred everything we disowned, until we were ready to own it again. However, as adults, many of us fail to do the work of owning it. **Shadow work, then, is the process of giving a productive outlet to the murky parts of ourselves. It is an exploration of the conscious mind, without judgment.** The only way to fix our dark-natured problems is to bring them into the light.

Examining our shadow side is a conscious process that allows us to accept and integrate the shadow side into ourselves. We confront trauma and pain head on, so that they lose their power over us. When we learn to accept and embrace our perceived shortcomings, we will no longer be controlled by them. The aim is to harness the energy of the shadow, not destroy it, in order to heal.

Acknowledging and integrating the shadow is one of the clearest pathways to living a meaningful, authentic life. Without shadow work, the healing we do is fractional. Whatever we deny in ourselves we project onto others. By integrating our shadow into our whole selves, we will heal not only our inner wounds but also our relationships.

When we treat our shadow as our best friend rather than the enemy we're used to avoiding, we begin the journey back to wholeness—our truest, highest self. This is shadow work at its core: facing *the entirety* of our own soul. As Carl Jung said, "Everyone carries a shadow, and the less it is embodied in the individual's conscious life, the blacker and denser it is." Embodiment of our shadow, then, is the key. The true secret of the spiritual warrior is not avoidance—it's authenticity.

"Shadow work is the process of addressing the pains and traumas within. Confronting the fears head on, they lose their power. It is ultimately an act of embracing more love by knowing the divine wisdom and perfection of every situation."

—*Andye Murphy*

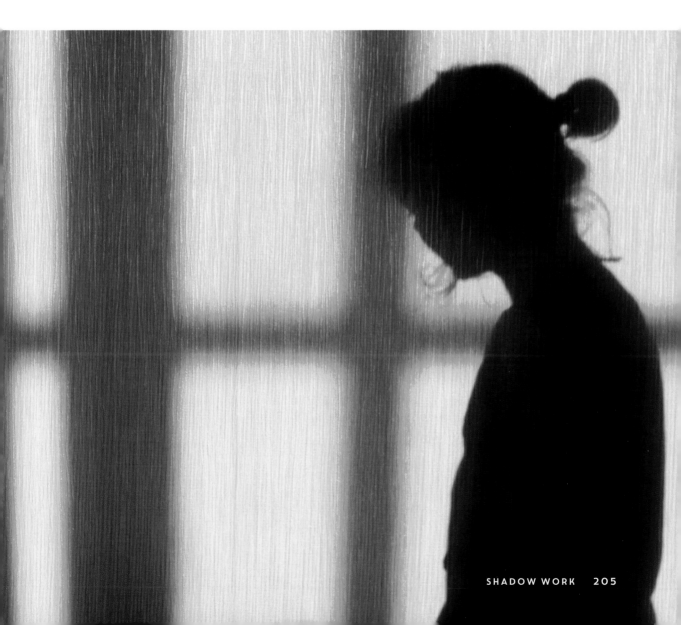

THE SHADOW ARCHETYPES

Some Jungian philosophers claim there are four main archetypes of the subconscious mind: the king, which represents wisdom, safety, and order; the warrior, which represents energy, loyalty, and honor; the magician, which represents secrets and the inner world; and the lover, which represents the senses, passion, and beauty. In their highest forms, these archetypes represent the best attributes of mature and integrated adulthood. Each of these archetypes also has two shadow sides: one that is active, and one that is passive.

ARCHETYPE	SHADOW SIDE: ACTIVE	SHADOW SIDE: PASSIVE
King	Tyrant	Weakling
Warrior	Sadist	Masochist
Magician	Manipulator	Innocent One
Lover	Addicted Lover	Impotent Lover

The goal of understanding the archetypes and their shadow sides is to learn how they operate within you. The shadow archetypes can help you identify thoughts and behavioral patterns that are connected to your shadow side, and therefore can bring about negative feelings and unhealthy actions. Shadow work helps you bring these shadow archetypes into the light and integrate them so that they can be expressed in their highest form. So, for instance, if your shadow harbors the tyrant king, you could work on transforming demanding, tyrannical impulses into wisdom that protects and keeps others safe.

Ways to Do Shadow Work

Because we've buried our shadows deep in our subconscious minds, it can be tricky to identify them. Here are some exercises that are helpful.

JOURNALING

Journaling is one of the most effective ways to bring the dark sides of ourselves into the light for analysis and integration. Here are some shadow work prompts to get you started:

- In what ways do I feel I act inauthentically? Why?
- In what ways do I lie to people? Why?
- What am I in denial of in my own life? Why?
- What is the biggest promise I have broken to someone else? Do I regret it?
- What is the biggest promise I have broken to myself? Do I regret it?
- What are some emotions that I try to avoid? Why do I do that?
- What are my bad habits? Why do I keep them?
- What is my biggest regret? What decision would I have made instead?
- In what ways do I feel unloved by other people? Why?
- In what ways do I feel unloved by myself? Why?

"Perhaps all the dragons of our lives are princesses who are only waiting to see us once beautiful and brave. Perhaps everything terrible is in its deepest being something helpless that wants help from us."

—*Rainer Maria Rilke*

INTEGRATING YOUR SOUL MAGIC

With all the ancient healing techniques outlined in this book, you might be eager to unleash all of your soul's magic! Take your time. Integration of these powerful and life-changing modalities will take practice and patience, but doing so will help you express and access your soul's true magic.

Trust your intuition and choose a few modalities that call to you and/or compliment each other. Then go deep and get inspired! You'll find that when you surrender to a new modality, it will awaken you to new experiences. You may be covered in chills while reading or practicing, have prophetic knowings that begin to pop into your mind, suddenly meet your spirit guides or loved ones in a dream, or even realize that you've clearly discovered your life purpose. Let new paths unfold before you and follow them to new destinations. Reach out to like-minded friends and community as you experiment.

While exploring your timeless soul, always remember that you are in control of your life. Not the stars, past lives, spirit guides, angels, ancestors, or tarot cards. All of these are tools to help you navigate your best life, but you are the captain of your own ship and you steer with your own free will. We hope you use this book as a map on your journey and say yes to all the places you want to go.

More than anything, remember to have fun on this grand adventure! We are meant to play on Earth with joy and reverence. Having fun brings our most authentic self forward to light up the world. If it isn't fun for you, it isn't for you—period. Let joy be your guide and we promise you'll always be led exactly to the people, places, and events that bring out your soul's brightest and most powerful magic!

Love, light, and black holes,
Arizona Bell and Morgan Garza